XXL:
OBESITY AND THE LIMITS OF SHAME

Obese individuals are twice as likely to experience heart failure as non-obese people. More than 85 per cent of Type 2 diabetes sufferers are overweight. In the United States, obese and overweight individuals make up more than two-thirds of the adult population. Public health organizations and governments have traditionally tried to combat obesity through shame-inducing policies, which assure people that they can easily lose weight by eating right and exercising. This generic approach has failed, as it does little to address the personal, genetic, and cultural challenges faced by obese individuals.

XXL directly confronts the global public health sector by proposing an innovative, alternative policy – the 'healthy living voucher' – for decreasing high calorie consumption and its related health problems. Neil Seeman and Patrick Luciani argue that many public health campaigns have made the problem of obesity worse by minimizing how difficult it is for individuals to lose weight. XXL challenges governments to abandon top-down planning solutions in favour of bottom-up innovations to confront the obesity crisis.

(University of Toronto Centre for Public Management Monograph Series on Public Policy and Public Administration)

NEIL SEEMAN is director of the Health Strategy Innovation Cell and a senior resident in health system innovation at Massey College, University of Toronto.

PATRICK LUCIANI is a senior resident at Massey College, University of Toronto.

The University of Toronto Centre for Public Management Monograph Series

Editor: Andrew Stark, University of Toronto
Funder: The Donner Canadian Foundation

The University of Toronto Centre for Public Management Monograph Series is an ongoing series of books on important topical matters in public administration and public policy that will engage not only the academic community but also policy- and opinion-makers in Canada and elsewhere.

Books are included in the series based on their originality, capacity to provoke public debate, and academic rigour.

For a list of books published in the series, see page 163.

NEIL SEEMAN AND PATRICK LUCIANI

XXL

Obesity and the Limits of Shame

University of Toronto Centre for Public Management Monograph Series

© University of Toronto Press Incorporated 2011
Toronto Buffalo London
www.utppublishing.com
Printed in Canada

ISBN 978-0-7727-8628-9 (cloth)
ISBN 978-0-7727-8627-2 (paper)

Printed on acid-free, 100% post-consumer recycled paper with
vegetable-based inks.

Library and Archives Canada Cataloguing in Publication

Seeman, Neil
XXL : obesity and the limits of shame / Neil Seeman and Patrick Luciani.

(University of Toronto Centre for Public Management monograph series)
Includes bibliographical references and index.
ISBN 978-0-7727-8628-9 (bound). – ISBN 978-0-7727-8627-2 (pbk.)

1. Obesity – Government policy.   2. Obesity – Economic aspects.
3. Obesity – Psychological aspects.   I. Luciani, Patrick   II. Title.
III. Series: University of Toronto Centre for Public Management
monograph series

RA645.O23S43 2011   362.196'398   C2011-900674-X

Produced for the University of Toronto Centre for Public Management by
the University of Toronto Press.

Contents

Foreword

Obesity, as Neil Seeman and Patrick Luciani argue in *XXL*, is not only a public health 'crisis.' It is a crisis for 'public health' – for the doctrines and protocols of that field.

The very term 'public health' implies approaches to our well-being that, far from being tailored to the needs of each of us as individuals, are meant to aid large numbers: the public as a whole. Its very essence impels it in the direction of one-size-fits-all measures. Hence, in dealing with obesity, public health officials have exhorted us to exercise, recommended changes to food labelling, advocated the banning of trans fats in restaurant food, issued dietary guidelines, and set forth exercise recommendations, all of which – as the authors note with keen insight – rely at one level on shaming the people they are trying to help.

Each of these efforts is meant to be useful to the public as a whole. None, fundamentally, has worked. A few have even been dangerously counterproductive, contributing to a climate in which impossible body images become aspirational.

Public health approaches have been flummoxed, the authors argue, because obesity is a deeply individual problem, one that manifests itself uniquely in each case. Genes, stress, hormones, portion sizes, the environment, commuting and fast food, depression and comfort food, sedentary lifestyles and snack food: all play a causal role, but in each person the mix is different.

And so then should be the appropriate treatment. Of the innumerable exercise and diet regimes available, and the options for surgery and lifestyle changes, and the contributions that can be made by psychotherapy and pharmaceuticals, each individual requires his or her own tailored combination to deal with his or her own unique condition.

In the face of this reality, what is 'public health' to do? The authors offer an innovative answer. Borrowing an instrument used by other public policy domains – education, welfare, housing – when the need is to enable individuals to find their own solutions to complex policy problems, they recommend a 'healthy living' voucher. Each individual, in consultation with his or her primary care provider, would use it to create a bespoke regimen, mixing, matching, and experimenting to find 'whatever works.'

This is public health for the twenty-first century. *XXL* is compelling, original, lucid, engagingly written, anecdote-filled, data-driven, and – above all – deeply sympathetic, to both public health officials and private individuals wrestling with weight issues. I am pleased to have the opportunity – and grateful, as always, to the Donner Canadian Foundation for providing the means – to publish *XXL* in the University of Toronto Centre for Public Management Monograph Series.

Andrew Stark
Editor
University of Toronto Centre for Public Management Monograph Series

Acknowledgments

We are grateful to our peer reviewers and their valuable comments. Special thanks are due to the research assistance of Mr Wendell Adjetey, to whom we are greatly indebted. Finally, we thank our editor, Andrew Stark of the University of Toronto, especially for his wisdom on the reality vs theory of public policy.

All errors or omissions are our own. We are students of obesity – and human complexity.

Neil Seeman and Patrick Luciani

XXL:
OBESITY AND THE LIMITS OF SHAME

Introduction: The Genesis of Shame

Shaming is an attempt to keep people from transgressing by invoking public disgrace. What does shame have to do with obesity?

If you majored in English literature, you will recall *Beowulf*, the eighth-century Anglo-Saxon war epic with some thirty-two hundred lines of verse. Beowulf, nephew of King Hygelac of the Geats, battles bloodied and bare-fisted against three foes: the monster Grendel, who takes perverse pleasure in murdering innocents; Grendel's mother; and, after his heroic return to Geatland, a fire-breathing dragon. The dragon, enraged because a mere man has managed to steal a goblet from his treasure, ravages the land. Beowulf ventures forth to slay the dragon, but his men, except for the young Wiglaf, desert him.

Beowulf, with the gods gazing upon him in judgment, grunts in Gaelic as he presses ahead: 'No he ære feohyfte for sceotendum scamian orfte!' Or, in modern English: 'I shall shame you, you bastards!' Beowulf suffers a fatal blow, and at his funeral, Wiglaf publicly shames his companions for their cowardice.

And there you have it: the earliest known literary reference to the use of the verb 'shame' (Old English, *scamian*) as a method of exacting punishment – a hero's battle cry that serves to humiliate his men for eternity.

Today, obesity policy is still to use shame to punish and humiliate. Jon Leibowitz, chairman of the Federal Trade Commission, has committed his agency to 'shaming companies that aren't doing enough' to 'voluntarily' combat obesity. Shame is an increasingly popular weapon in the armamentarium of public health. It is wielded by generals and managers and CEOs; and by parents to set limits and to civilize. Shame and embarrassment work remarkably well to change children's behaviour. Ancient Greeks distinguished shame in the sense of 'dishonour' (*aiskhyne*) from shame in the sense of 'modesty' (*aidos*). Public health bureaucrats, whose job, they feel, is to modify behaviour, think of shame in the former sense, as a policy weapon to dishonour those who, by their actions, facilitate obesity and those who, in their eyes, are guilty of the crime of being obese. In the past, they used the same weapon, with varying success, to address the great public health challenges of our time: smoking, alcoholism, and unsafe sex.

The first modern English reference to shaming came in 1534, in a bizarre letter describing monastic life and activities in the early Tudor period. An archdeacon, shocked that two brothers, Whytford and Little, were soliciting nuns for sexual service during confession, said of Whytford: 'He hath a brazen forehed, which shameth at nothing.' Thus, it seems, was born the modern phrase, 'He has no shame.' How many times have you seen a 'zaftig' person wolfing down potato chips or cookies in public and thought to yourself, 'Doesn't she have any shame?'

To be brazen has always been connected with public shame; in *Roman Forgeries and Christian Ethics*, Crashaw refers in 1606 to the 'brazen face of the whore of Babylon, who shames with no sin.' To be brazen is to be loud and clamorous (as a brass band); James Joyce later described the 'brazen clashes of the soldiers' band.' One who is shamed cannot hide because his face betrays him. Annibale Pocaterra, a sixteenth-century physician and poet, in a book-length study on shame, *Due Dialogi della Vergogna* (Two Dialogues on Shame), wrote that shame threatens the soul. Its signs appear on the face 'like a flash of fire.'

'Thou sing'st not in the day, as shaming any eye should thee behold,' wrote William Shakespeare, in the 1594 narrative poem *The Rape of Lucrece*. Lucretia, in Roman legend, was the daughter of Spurius Lucretius, prefect of Rome, and the wife of Tarquinius Collatinus. After Lucretia is raped by Sextus, the King's violent son, she admits to her dishonour in public – before her father, her husband, her brother Brutus, and their kinsmen. She then stabs herself to death in humiliation. In revenge for her shame, Brutus leads an uprising that destroys the Tarquin monarchy and establishes the Roman republic. Two policy messages emerge. The first is that shame is destructive, a widely known trigger to despair and self-harm. Its consequences are brutal. The second message is that out of its ashes something better can emerge.

This book is about the failure of the culture of shame to help in the battle against obesity. Far from helping, it has led to a rise in depression, anxiety, and self-loathing. This book suggests a better way.

1 The Paradoxical Costs of Fat

In Springfield, Illinois, Field House Pizza and Pub owner Tom Hart boasts: 'We made something very unhealthy even unhealthier.' He's talking about his 'Shoe Burrito,' a new, cheesier twist on the eighty-two-year-old classic 'Horseshoe,' 2,700 calories for $7.75. In Springfield and cities like it across America, six hundred thousand people signed up for the 2010 Denny's 'Grand Slam for a Year' promotion.[1] For this all-you-can-eat contest, each entrant gets to order fifty-two servings of a Denny's 'Grand Slam' breakfast, or two eggs, two bacon strip links, two grease-soaked sausages, and two thick pancakes. That's a total of 44,824 calories. Most contestants cannot eat this much, of course – more than thirty-seven days of recommended calories for an adult woman at one sitting – so they bring their friends. It's like a tailgate party without the football.

Like TV's lovable Homer Simpson from the show's fictional city of 'Springfield,' contestants boast – nowadays on social media sites like Facebook – about their participation in 'extreme eating' sports like the Grand Slam. One Russian pancake-gorging winner died during an all-you-can-eat contest in March 2009 before being able to collect his reward. The British media were all over the story.

So, some might ask, 'Do these people have no shame?' Are Denny's contestants aware of the health consequences of their behaviour? Do they even stop to *think* that others, including those whose opinions mean the most to them, perceive their behaviour as grotesque? Their spouse may well say, as Marge Simpson tells Homer one day: 'I'm finding myself less attracted to you.'

In one episode of *The Simpsons*, Homer, who normally weighs in at over two hundred pounds, balloons outwards (to three hundred pounds), and as a consequence, like tens of thousands of other North American adults, he loses out on sex. 'We found a 2.5-fold difference in risk of erectile dysfunction when we compared obese men who did little exercise with men who were not overweight and averaged 30 minutes of vigorous exercise a day,'[2] says Eric Rimm, associate professor of epidemiology and nutrition at the Harvard School of Public Health. The more weight a person puts on, the less drawn he is to sex. Food is where the craving lies. Shifting around excess weight makes sex too difficult, too strenuous; vigorous activity is just too tiring. Bulky people worry, too, that their partners will no longer find them desirable; and this is true. 'I say "no" before he gets a chance to say "no,"' one overweight woman complains anonymously online. 'That way, I don't get my feelings hurt.' He, equally fat, may be saying 'no' because of muted desire or perhaps because he can't. 'In our study population, we found that lower testosterone levels and diminished ratings for sexual quality of life were correlated with increased body mass index,'[3] says Dr Ahmad Hammoud of the University of Utah and lead author of a study exploring this taboo topic, one of the many costs of obesity. The corollaries of fat have many dimensions, many of which we're just learning about – poor health, reduced quality of life, low self-esteem, babies born with defects, loss of productivity and longevity, and a huge financial burden on society.

Obesity and Quality of Life

Weight interferes not only with one's sex life and marriage, but also with many other humdrum aspects of life. In September 2002 a reporter noticed that former Vice-President Al Gore's left ring finger was bare. Had he and Tipper split up? No, he assured the crowd at the Brookings Institution in Washington later that month. He had gained so much weight that he could no longer slip the ring on. (Eight years later, he and his wife did announce that they would divorce; there's no evidence his changing girth was to blame.) A ring that doesn't fit is a small embarrassment to be sure, but small embarrassments add up. Weight can limit your ability to work, to move, to provide care for those you love. The classic measure of quality of life is what scientists call a QALY (pronounced 'Kalee'), or 'Quality Adjusted Life Year.' A recent study from the Mailman School of Public Health and Nursing at Columbia University looked at the QALYs associated with the two greatest public health hazards in the Western world, which are smoking and obesity.[4] Smoking had a bigger impact on mortality (loss of life) than on morbidity (illness), whereas it was the other way around for obesity. You die from cigarettes; you suffer more from obesity. Because of the strik- ing increase in obesity rates in recent years, obesity now contributes at least as much as smoking to the global burden of disease. Being obese comes not as a single spy, but with a full battalion of ills: hip pain, knee ache, huffing and puffing, bed wetting, and a host of major and minor insults that make life uncomfortable. Elvis Presley, whose weight shot up toward the end of his life, once found himself in a difficult situation while bumping and grinding on stage. As he explained to his worship- ful audience, his extra poundage had split the seat of his jumpsuit. His career fizzled after that, though his legacy (the image is always of a youthful and slim Elvis) survives.

Obesity and Self-Esteem

Social stigma – being made to feel an outcast – shames the person who is targeted. The actress Kate Winslet had difficulty managing her weight when she was an adolescent. She started her acting career when she was sixteen and at that point weighed 185 pounds and was nicknamed 'Blubber.' 'I was bullied for being chubby,' she says. Chub- by children are twice as likely as slim children to say their self-esteem is low. They're sadder, lonelier, and more nervous than other chil- dren as well as more likely, it turns out, to turn for solace to alcohol and drugs. Heavy children feel they are incompetent when it comes to athletics; they think they look bad, and they don't do well making friends. They're ashamed of their appearance so they don't look you in the eye or smile comfortably or make the first move to get to know you. In the early years, kids don't notice much, but social acceptance declines after adolescence when teenagers become very body con- scious. But, in what was a surprise to us, not all research confirms this fact. A number of studies have examined the supposed link between weight and self-esteem, and they don't all agree. Some find no connec- tion, and that is a mystery to obesity researchers. Why the contradic- tions? The more you explore the field of obesity, the more you realize that it is dizzyingly contradictory. As we'll see throughout this book, people who struggle with weight, and many smart people who study weight issues for a living, hold different points of view and arrive at very different data-driven conclusions about obesity's cause and impact.

'Body Mass Index' and Pregnancy

How do we measure weight? Usually by an old and crude measurement tool called the body mass index, or BMI, calculated by dividing a person's weight in kilograms by their height in metres and then dividing the total by their height in metres. Being overweight today has historically been defined as a BMI of over 27.3 for adult women and over 27.8 for men. A BMI of over 30 is considered obese. The late Senator Ted Kennedy had a BMI of 34.2. Marlon Brando's, toward the end, was 44.3.

BMI is not the best measure of unhealthy weight. An important 2008 study found that BMI was extremely limited as a predictor of health risks.[5] A bulging waistline, it found, better predicts premature death than a person's BMI. The message: You're better off pear-shaped than apple-shaped. For a longitudinal study published in the *New England Journal of Medicine*, researchers tracked nearly 360,000 men and women in nine European countries over a decade. Participants in the study ranged in age from 25 to 70. Men with waists measuring over forty inches proved to be the ones at most risk. For women, the danger zone was a waistline of over thirty-five inches. Average waistlines in America have expanded by about one inch per decade since the 1960s. And more and more research shows that bigger bellies pose a greater risk of death, even for people who are in the 'normal' BMI zone.

For this book, especially in chapters 1 and 2, we rely heavily on statistics and research using the BMI measure simply because this is the (flawed) foundation upon which researchers have historically analysed obesity. Given the groundbreaking *NEJM* study on waist size and risk, our references to BMI studies should therefore be viewed with a critical eye, which itself underscores what we see as the severe limitations of the current body of scientific knowledge about the causes and potential cures for obesity.

Extra weight, as calculated by BMI, is a risk factor for pregnant women and leads to sicker babies and more difficult pregnancies. The consequences can include spontaneous miscarriage, gestational diabetes (diabetes that develops in pregnant women and reverts to normal at the end of pregnancy), pre-eclampsia (high blood pressure during pregnancy, with protein in the urine), Caesarean delivery, venous thromboembolism (blood clots), and infant congenital defects. This is critically important to know for public health policy because most women gain more weight than they should during pregnancy. The medical community's focus in the West has been on preventing premature babies, but increasing evidence shows that high-weight babies face health challenges in later life. 'A pregnant woman should have her weight monitored regularly during pregnancy at all antenatal appointments with midwives, GPs and obstetricians, because every risk of pregnancy, both to the mother and to the baby, is increased with maternal obesity,'[6] Dr David Haslam, the UK's National Obesity Forum chairman, told *The Observer* in January 2010. About 30 per cent of pregnant women are obese; and 35 per cent of women who die in childbirth are obese. Obesity during pregnancy is a serious matter. It affects not only the mother but the children as well. And as pregnant women get larger, so too do future generations.

Obesity and Cancer

For any adult with severe obesity – we call them 'XXLs' because of the size of clothes they need to wear – there is a high mortality risk for cancers of the esophagus, colon and rectum, liver, breast, uterus, ovaries, gallbladder, kidney, and pancreas. In the U.S., excess weight is linked to 90,000 cancer deaths annually.[7] Also in the U.S., 14 per cent of deaths from cancer in men, and 20 per cent in women, are an indirect or direct result of overweight or obesity. Yet only about 3 per cent of all new cancer *diagnoses* are thought to result directly from obesity. That's hard to understand, but as we will see again and again, there are many paradoxes in the field of obesity. Breast cancer risk, for instance, depends on whether a woman has or has not reached menopause. Before menopause, obese women have a *lower* risk of developing breast cancer than other women. After menopause, obese women have one-and-a-half times the risk of other women. Scientists estimate that 11,000 to 18,000 deaths per year from breast cancer in American women over age fifty could be avoided if women were able to maintain a BMI under 25 as they aged.[8] Gaining forty-five pounds or more after age eighteen doubles your chances of developing breast cancer after menopause. This pre- and post-menopause discrepancy is another indication that obesity is not an issue that lends itself to generalizations. Each person suffering from obesity has to be understood differently, depending on his or her biology and life circumstances.

For cancer of the uterus, obesity has been estimated to account for about 40 per cent of cases. If you are obese, your risk of cancer of the uterus is three to four times higher than normal. If your BMI is 34 or greater, your risk is more than six times higher. In prostate cancer, it's the more aggressive tumours that are linked to obesity, not the more common, slow-growth ones. Obesity in women has a stronger relationship to kidney cancer than obesity in men. The biological mechanisms by which obesity leads to cancer are, scientists think, different for different cancers. Possible triggers include changes in sex hormones because sex hormones are synthesized in fatty tissues. Cancers caused by obesity now pose an urgent threat to mankind and must be tackled immediately,[9] warns Sir Michael Marmot, Professor of Public Health at University College London. 'It's enormous, it's catastrophic,' he has said. 'The numbers are just frightening on a global scale.'

Type 2 Diabetes

There are three types of diabetes: Type 1, Type 2, and gestational. Type 1 diabetes is not linked to obesity and occurs when the 'islet cells' in the pancreas stop producing insulin. Type 2 and gestational diabetes are both conditions where the body does produce insulin but the response to insulin is impaired. Gestational diabetes is linked to hormonal changes during pregnancy. Type 2 diabetes is closely associated with obesity. Since 1990, there has been a 76 per cent rise in Type 2 diabetes in U.S. adults over thirty. *Quit Digging Your Grave with a Knife and Fork*[10] is a good guide to these issues, written by former Arkansas Governor Mike Huckabee, the Republican candidate for the presidency in 2008. Mr Huckabee lost over 110 pounds after his doctors informed him that he had Type 2 diabetes and would likely not live more than ten more years unless he lost weight. Gain eleven to eighteen pounds and you double your risk of diabetes. Gain forty-four pounds and you quadruple it. A BMI greater than 35 makes your risk seven times as high as that of your lean neighbour.

Weight put on in childhood is tied to Type 2 diabetes in adulthood. Type 2 diabetes was once an adult disease; but obese children around the world are increasingly developing this kind of diabetes. Too many fat cells undermine insulin sensitivity so that sugar, instead of being converted into energy, gets released into the bloodstream. That's because fat cells secrete hormones such as adiponectin and resistin that cause the body to resist insulin.[11]

Hypertension and Stroke

If you're obese, your blood pressure is twice as likely as otherwise to be high. If you're severely obese (with a BMI over 40), the risk shoots up four times. High blood pressure (*hypertension*) is the most significant known risk factor for *stroke*, and central (around the middle) fat distribution (more so than BMI) correlates closely with both. Obese children are at risk for hypertension and cardiovascular illness when they become adults; but, interestingly, it is now clear that this is more often the case if they have a specific variant of a particular gene: the insulin-like growth factor type II (IGF-II). In other words, obesity is a risk factor for high blood pressure and for stroke, but these risks depend substantially on your individual genetic make-up.[12]

Heart Disease

Obesity is an independent risk factor for heart disease. This means that it can predispose you to heart problems even if you have no other risk factors. Obesity puts pounds on the heart by laying down fat deposits. Autopsy results show that the coronary arteries in obese people are teeming with atherosclerosis and fatty streaks. Obesity also injures the heart by raising blood pressure, increasing inflammation, making blood more likely to clot, and interfering with the lungs' ability to breathe. Being overweight and obese is associated with cardiac complications such as coronary heart disease, heart failure, and sudden death.[13] A case in point is the life story of John Candy, the Canadian comic actor. Candy struggled with obesity throughout his adult life. During the late 1980s and early 1990s he gained a large amount of additional weight, which, in a way, benefited his career: he was funny without having to work at it. The 'funny fat man' persona led to nearly forty feature films. What most fans did not know is that he struggled to lose weight, switching from diet to diet and trainer to trainer, from jogging to biking to swimming. When he turned forty, he began suffering from panic attacks. 'He would just stand backstage before he went on with his eyes shut, breathing in and out,' says producer Peter Kaminsky. These may have been the first signs of heart disease. At six a.m. on 4 March 1994, while on location in Mexico filming *Wagons East*, the forty-three-year-old Candy suffered a heart attack and died in his sleep.

Gall Bladder Disease

Obesity, especially in women, brings with it gallstones and gall bladder disease. Oddly, however, thinner men have more complicated gall bladder disease than do fatter men. On the other hand, over one-quarter of all the days in hospital for gall bladder disease in middle-aged women can be linked to obesity, which is another great obesity paradox.[14] Only if you're a woman does obesity, on average, double your chances of developing gallstones.

Knee and Hip Pain

Obesity is one of the main risk factors for osteoarthritis. Overweight women have nearly four times the risk of arthritis of the knee; for overweight men, the risk is five times greater. For many years the association between obesity and osteoarthritis had been attributed simply to the effects of overload on weight-bearing joints; more recently, though, it has been understood that osteoarthritis is the result of complex interactions of genetic, metabolic, hormonal, and biomechanical factors that make hips and knees vulnerable to heavy loads.[15] For every two pounds you gain, your risk of osteoarthritis goes up 9 to 13 per cent.

Breathing

Evidence is mounting that obesity is also a risk factor for asthma – especially among the poor, for reasons unknown.[16] Just one high-fat meal like a Denny's Grand Slam has been shown to increase cholesterol and lead to inflammation of the lungs. Heart attacks after big bacon, pancake, and sausage breakfasts are not uncommon, especially if an obese person already at risk rises suddenly from a sitting position. Later in the day, obesity is also associated with what doctors call 'obstructive sleep apnea,' which itself leads to many health problems, especially brain problems and heart disease.

Urinary Incontinence

Urinary incontinence, often humiliating to those affected, is a common affliction, particularly in older women. It causes varying degrees of unintended urine 'leakage,' especially when coughing or straining or laughing or whenever you're excited or frightened. Obesity has long been known to increase the risk of urinary incontinence, probably because of increased pressure on the bladder. Losing weight significantly reduces the severity of this embarrassing symptom.[17]

Loss of Libido

Many overweight men are interested in sex but are seldom up to the task. Nearly 80 per cent of men who report erectile dysfunction (ED) are overweight or obese. ED is also associated with Type 2 diabetes. Abdominal obesity may contribute to ED due to an increased inflammatory response, or due to reduced testosterone levels, both of which reduce blood flow to the penis.[18] Is there any relation between obesity and penis size? No, but being obese can give the illusion that your penis is smaller than it used to be. Obese men develop a fat pad at the base of the penis, and when the penis is flaccid, it retracts into this fat pad. Obese men, XXLs, are often not able to see their penis without the aid of a mirror, since their chest and stomach block the view. What has been called the 'genital view' test is a simple if humiliating way of testing for obesity, for both men and women: patients are asked whether they can see their genitals by looking straight down. We estimate that at least 10 per cent of the Western population would now flunk this test.

Bullying and Obesity

Obese children, especially boys, are likely to be victims of bullying. Overweight children report significantly more verbal and physical bullying than their thinner classmates,[19] as we saw with Kate Winslet. However, it is incorrect to say that obesity is always a social problem for all children and that all heavy children at all ages are ostracized or left out of the in-crowd. Anti-obesity public health campaigns can sometimes exaggerate the problem of bullying and may even contribute to it by drawing attention to something that children might otherwise solve on their own. Obese children can sometimes be the bullies, too: bullying by children is a complex psychological phenomenon rooted in the perpetrator's own lowered self-esteem.

Drugs and Alcohol

Because alcohol contains on average seven calories per gram, there is a good chance that alcoholics will become obese; oddly, though, obese men are not especially prone to substance abuse. On the other hand, there are definite links in young adult women among depression, obesity, and alcohol abuse – yet another indication that overweight people differ widely in their proclivities. 'For women there is a great deal of overlap between these common emotional and health problems that span early adulthood,'[20] says Carolyn McCarty, the lead author of a recent study published in a psychiatry journal. Actress Kate Hudson lost twenty pounds for a film she was making. She didn't go on any particular diet or fitness program. She did only one thing – she stopped drinking. 'I love my glass of wine. I love tequila,' said the glamorous, wide-eyed Ms Hudson, but she stopped, and it worked. A new study of 19,220 U.S. women, however, shows that normal-weight women drinking light to moderate amounts of alcohol gain *less* weight and have *less* risk for obesity than non-drinkers over the long term – again, a paradoxical study result.[21]

Depression and Anxiety

Where obesity is most studied is in connection with depression and anxiety. The Canadian Community Health Survey, the gold standard survey on the health behaviours of Canadians, examined adults twenty to sixty-four years old and found that obesity was significantly associated with mood disorders but not with anxiety disorders.[22] This is puzzling, since depression and anxiety usually go together in most scientific studies. But much is counter-intuitive about obesity research. Many U.S. studies have found an association between depression and obesity in men, but not in women, while many studies outside the U.S. have not found *any* connection between obesity and depression. Some studies have found the association particularly strong for teenage girls. One group found a 25 per cent increase in the odds of having either a mood disorder or an anxiety disorder if you were obese.[23] Another study concluded that BMI is associated with depression in women, but that abdominal obesity is linked to depression in both women and men.[24]

These perplexing, often conflicting public health findings from the best researchers in the world highlight the importance of taking many factors into account when assessing the risks of obesity – gender, but also sociodemographic characteristics and personality factors. Obese individuals as a group tend to score high on various psychiatric dimensions of depression, such as anhedonia (not being able to feel pleasure), alexithymia (not being able to put a name to your emotions), external locus of control (feeling under the sway of others), impulsivity, and interpersonal dependency (not being able to make decisions, leaning on others).[25] Whatever the reasons, obesity does increase the risk for individuals to claim disability pensions on the basis of psychiatric disorders, and this is one way by which it imposes a large financial cost on society.[26]

Length of Life

Obesity causes approximately 350,000 excess deaths a year in the United States, deaths that could be prevented if we had a public policy that helped people make better decisions about what, how much, and how often they eat and what they can do to keep physically active. Men with body mass indices over 40 give up about twenty years of life. Because they tend to store their fat in their thighs rather than in their stomachs, women have a better relationship to obesity. Women with equally high BMIs lose only five years of life.

Those who have lost loved ones to XXL-related illness such as heart disease and weight-related cancers know the real costs of obesity at first hand; as do those who have lost children to weight-related pregnancy problems; and those who themselves suffer from weight-related arthritis and breathing problems. The intriguing part for us as writers and as researchers is the mismatch between, on the one hand, people's basic knowledge of the dire medical consequences of obesity – which are well-known within all public health bureaucracies of today's Western governments – and effective corrective policy – which seems to elude all nations, wealthy or poor.

What is the policy solution? That is the focus of this book. Debates over 'for profit' versus 'socialized medicine' are mostly irrelevant to this issue. We call them public policy sideshows. To get serious about obesity and its consequences, policy makers need to focus less on tinkering with the funding formula for physicians and hospitals and more on stopping people from scarfing down bags upon bags of potato chips. Nowhere in the world is there a working 'system model' to push back on obesity. People may be thinner in some geographic areas than in others, but it's not because of a health care 'system' or a government or employer insurance scheme. Real solutions hang on the successful introduction of policy incentives that allow people to choose from among as many credible options as possible and find one that works for them. As we will see, such incentives can be implemented in any system of health care in the Western world. Though we are Canadians living in a public Medicare system, we are neither for nor against a public system as such. Nor are we passing judgment here on private markets in health care, as one sees in Singapore ('Medisave,' which allows Singaporeans to put aside income in a Medisave account to meet future personal hospitalization or outpatient expenses). We care only about what works to prevent and combat obesity.

The Productivity Costs of Obesity

Obesity affects us all since, even if we are thin, we pay into the health care costs of managing obesity. The annual financial cost of adult obesity alone in the U.S. in 2006 was estimated at $147 billion, at least 6 per cent of all health care costs – possibly as high as 10 per cent or even 20 per cent, depending on what you include in the bucket. Today, four years after these most recent CDC data, the costs have undoubtedly shot up. The slope of this cost curve will be increasing sharply, given that one in three U.S. children is now overweight or obese. The cost of lost productivity is high: $12.8 billion in annual losses to U.S. businesses from absenteeism; $30 billion annually due to reduced productivity on the job; and at least $35 billion spent every year on weight loss products and weight loss services. People who are fat take more time off work, equivalent in the U.S. to twenty-two days of lost production per year, according to the 2009 U.S. Annual Obesity Society's conference. The obese pay with their lives; the rest of society, including thin people (and their employers), pay with their pocketbooks. It has been estimated (using CDC data) that the average obese person in the U.S. spent $1,429 more on medical costs in 2006 than a normal-weight person.

Obesity matters for innovation and enterprise. It is in nobody's interest to have huge swaths of the industrialized world's labour supply breathing hard after a fifteen- or twenty-minute walk. A 2009 study looked at 370 recruits for firefighting and emergency medic jobs in Boston and found that almost all were either overweight or obese (almost half the recruits, 42 per cent, failed the required treadmill exercise test).[27] Nor is it of benefit for our planet that so many with such creative promise – intellectual, artistic, technical – are at risk of being eradicated by heart attack or premature stroke in their forties, just as they're reaching their creative peak. All but the most isolated among us know the medical risks, but many of us behave as if we were oblivious; we run on autopilot, enjoying the here-and-now of pleasurable consumption, inured to the cacophony of public health messages telling us how we've got to 'get moving' and 'eat healthy foods.' We tune out.

Our own research bears this out. According to Google Trends™, global news references to obesity have been edging ever upwards over the past five years. Searching about 15 million books published from 1800 to 2008, using data from Google's Ngram Viewer application, we discovered that literary and policy references to obesity shot upward after 1960. The major media, by reporting daily on obesity research, tell us that much of the world is now considerably overweight or obese. We all know this, if not in as much detail as obesity researchers do. Reporters keep writing about how fat we all are. But paradoxically, when a big news story on obesity does break, public interest in the issue doesn't rise – it either doesn't budge or actually declines. We're fatigued by fat news.

It is, of course, possible to be hefty and healthy. Many Internet bloggers and cocktail party contrarians like to say this. All of which raises the question of how best to attack an obesity crisis that affects different people in very different ways. In a 2008 study led by the University of Michigan's MaryFran Sowers, 51 per cent of overweight adults – roughly 36 million people across the United States – were found to have mostly normal levels of blood pressure, cholesterol, blood fats called triglycerides, and blood sugar.[28] Almost one-third of obese (BMI over 30) adults – nearly 20 million people – also fell into this healthy range, meaning that either none or only one of the above measures was 'abnormal.' At the same time, about one-quarter of adults in the recommended-weight range had unhealthy levels of at least two of these measures. That means that some 16 million healthy-weight individuals are at risk for the kinds of heart problems usually associated with obesity. Study co-author Judith Wylie-Rosett, a nutrition researcher at Albert Einstein College of Medicine in New York, warned that the study shouldn't send the message 'that we don't need to worry about weight.' There's no room for complacency. We must try to understand obesity and we must try to develop a public policy that does justice to its complexity.

As a generation, today's North Americans are the first to face substantially more disability and disease than their parents did. This is remarkable in an age of prosperity. It is not because of any economic downturn. It is simply because we take in too many calories and expend too few. We may live longer than our parents, yet we will be unhealthier for longer due to obesity-related chronic disease. Chronic illnesses cost U.S. businesses $1.1 trillion annually in terms of productivity. A primary driver of chronic illness is obesity. Why? As we've just seen, obesity leads to higher blood pressure, to heart disease, and to diabetes; and problems stemming from other diseases mushroom when our bodies juggle too much weight. To make health care costs manageable in places like the United States, we need to get obesity rates down to 1998 levels, when only 19 per cent of Americans were obese. As of 2009, 26.7 per cent of U.S. adults nationwide were obese. Nineteen per cent still sounds like a lot, but those were the good old days. Only two jurisdictions – Colorado and Washington, DC – have obesity rates below 20 per cent today. Ten years ago, twenty-eight states had obesity rates below 20 per cent of their adult population. The U.S. Surgeon General in 2001 called for a federal public health initiative to reduce obesity to 15 per cent of the adult population – a goal that far eludes every state today. Public health programs have tried to slim us down, but they are failing us. The more we are told by the state to cut down and exercise, the fatter we seem to get. This book explores this public health policy conundrum and proposes a policy solution. Where has public health policy gone wrong?

Where's the Fat?

It's not just that there are pockets of fat here and there. It's pretty much everywhere. All U.S. state health systems, for example, are suffering, though some far more than others. Obesity rates range from 18.6 per cent in Colorado to 34.4 per cent in Mississippi. Mississippi is the U.S. South, and southern states, despite stern public health efforts to curb excess weight, are consistently at the top of the list of obese states, according to 2009 data from the Centers for Disease Control and Prevention.[29] Adult obesity rates increased in twenty-eight out of fifty states in 2009. According to the Trust for America's Health and the Robert Wood Johnson Foundation, ten out of eleven states with the highest rates are located in the South; Mississippi has the highest for the sixth year in a row. In 2008, adult obesity rose in almost half of all states (twenty-three out of fifty). Today, Alabama, Arkansas, Kentucky, Louisiana, Mississippi, Missouri, Oklahoma, Tennessee, and West Virginia lead the growth in waist size, with more than 30 per cent of adults in these regions in the XXL–XXXL weight categories. Those states have large populations of

African American and poor, rural residents – groups with generally high rates of obesity in America. The only good news from the 2009 Trust's Report: the adult obesity rate in the District of Columbia fell from 22.3 per cent in 2009 to 21.5 per cent in 2008 (note that the current CDC data, mentioned earlier, put the District, with Colorado, under 20 per cent). The trust's executive director, Jeffrey Levi, attributed the one-year, statistically minor decline partly 'to new recreation centers and pools, as well as increased opportunity for public transportation.' This can be questioned, because people who frequent recreation centres and public pools and those who take public transit are probably in better health to start with.

Public health observers credit the good health in Colorado to ubiquitous bike, hiking, and ski trails. Colorado is the slimmest U.S. state and has been slim for a long time. But healthy, sporty people tend to like to live in places like Boulder, Colorado, and Vancouver, British Columbia (Canada's sportiest province). Putting more hiking trails in Mississippi and Tennessee would likely accomplish little for the local obese population now living there. But it would attract more athletes from other states.

In thirty-one states, more than one-quarter of adults are obese, says the 2009 report from the Trust for America's Health and the Robert Wood Johnson Foundation, which is a major funder of public health research. All the reports we describe here indicate that no state had a statistically significant decline from the prior year. 'No state is doing well,' Mr Levi told reporters in 2007. 'We have seen a dramatic increase throughout the country. Poor nutrition and physical inactivity are robbing America of our health and productivity.'

New Jersey alone spent $2.3 billion on obesity-related illnesses in 2003, half of which was paid for by taxpayers through Medicare and Medicaid, according to a 2006 report by the State Department of Health and Senior Services.[30] The total direct and indirect cost of obesity-induced diabetes to Americans is over $200 billion each year – an average of $1,900 per American household. Diabetes contributes to more than 200,000 American deaths each year. And we are not only talking about elderly adults. The hospitalization of heavy children in the United States has ballooned in recent years, according to a 2009 study in the journal *Health Affairs*.[31] The number of hospitalizations of obese kids and teens, ages two to nineteen, nearly doubled between 1999 and 2005, climbing from 21,743 to 42,429. The associated costs for these hospitalizations increased from almost $126 million in 2001 to almost $238 million in 2005. Obese patients need more hospitalizations, more out-patient visits, and more drugs to keep them out of hospital. One study, after controlling for age, sex, and underlying chronic disease, found that a person with a BMI of 40 spent US$115 more on health care per year than a person with a BMI of 25.

The United States today spends $2.3 trillion per year on health care – almost twice as much per person as other industrialized nations. Are Americans getting what they pay for? Canada spends more than $180 billion on health care.[32] One of the great economic problems of our time is that health care dollars are too often squandered – in private health care systems, in public systems, and everywhere in between. About one-third of the health care dollars in First World countries are spent on treatments, drugs, and tests that don't actually improve health outcomes. In every industrialized country, health economists are warning that unless health systems eliminate needless spending and put health care dollars to better use, spiralling costs will undermine long-term fiscal security.

It's hard to project the future costs of obesity. No country is good at this kind of prediction because it is mostly guesswork, left to the domain of 'long-range scenario planners' who have little sense of what science will discover about obesity two to five years from now. Things could be far, far worse than they are today; but there is also always the faint hope that a surprise will come along to abruptly eliminate the fat epidemic, such as unexpected drug treatments or gene therapies or miracle vaccines that will swing the obesity epidemic around. Some scientists, for instance, think that a virus may be responsible for obesity and are hunting for anti-infective agents.

Perhaps, in some people, weight gain *is* caused by a virus. What we do know for certain is that obesity arises from different causes in different people and produces different effects in different people, much like a typical virus. Given the biological variability of obesity, individuals have diverse needs. What works and what doesn't is not the same for everyone. Because the causes differ, effective treatments will, we feel, always differ from one person to another. That is why, as we will argue, a one-for-all public health policy to combat obesity will never work. Any public health policy for obesity, to be effective, will need to find as many ways as possible to manage specific obesity problems, to nurture unique solutions that will engage obese and overweight people and help them maintain their determination to get fit.

The Social Costs of XXL in North America

XXL means two times large, or, quite simply, massive for a man or woman of any height. We had small, medium, and large sizes for many, many years, and now we have evolved to extra-extra-extra-large (XXXL). 'Bigger snacks mean bigger slacks,' goes the mantra. Were it not for the popularity of 'husky' wear and 'relaxed fit' jeans, many clothing retailers across North America would be in serious financial trouble. Makers of men's jeans are accommodating heavier bulges in clever, subtle ways. Levi Strauss & Co. has added room in the seat and thigh in its 'skinny jeans' for men. True Religion had what it called a 'four-way stretch' spandex material in its line of men's jeans. In a public relations move to convey an anti-obesity brand image, The Gap dropped XXL sizes for men in 2008 – but kept the offerings available online.

A billboard on a U.S. interstate highway, captured on a 2008 cover of an academic journal called *Healthcare Papers,* advertises 'Big Men's Clothing: Up to Size 12X Shirts & Size 84 Pants.' One of us argued in that issue of the journal for a 'post-partisan' approach to obesity, drawing on Barack Obama's own 2008 U.S. election rhetoric, suggesting that serious policy dialogue about the problem of obesity needs to acknowledge the extraordinarily complex issues that countries ought to address. This book is our attempt at a post-partisan approach that encourages choice. But our policy suggestion on how to curb obesity, as will be seen, differs greatly from that of the White House. Indeed, the message from the current White House when it comes to health policy is largely about offering the public *less* choice, with civil service appointees dictating – based on large-scale 'comparative effectiveness trials' – which obesity treatments and interventions are to be publicly supported and financed. This is troubling when it comes to obesity, since large human trials obscure important individual differences.

It is difficult to get an exact read on precisely how overweight the world is. People lie on surveys – by about 30 to 35 per cent of actual body weight. A better approach to survey-style measurement, we suggest, is to look at the search terms that millions of people type into Google (or other online search engines) every day. Tens of millions of people, each day, 'google' books and movies and other items that they want to purchase. Google Insights™ enables users to analyse search terms – to assess the popularity of searches relative to the total universe of possible search terms. The proportion of people searching for information on a particular topic – say, obesity – is therefore what statisticians call 'normalized' or 'scaled.' We found it revealing that around the world, people are increasingly interested in finding out information about the local availability of 'XXL' sizes. This is increasingly so (roughly double) at periods of peak buying, right at the end of the year, near Christmas. In other words, our hypothesis is that since 2004, there has been a jump each successive year in the proportion of people inquiring (via Google) into whether or not their local store carries size XXL attire. That's because there are spikes in global searches for 'XXL sizes' at the end of each shopping year.

We, the authors of this book, live and work in Canada. An estimated 11 million Canadians are overweight, and about half a million are severely obese and in need of an urgent solution to their problem. As noted before, the fat epidemic is eclipsing the smoking epidemic in disease burden. More and more observers feel that obesity is even worse for society than smoking. We're not absolutely convinced about that; suffice it to say that both are public health hazards. Recent research certainly suggests that obese teenagers are as likely to die prematurely as are heavy smokers. More important, one of these challenges (smoking) is on an ongoing decline, while the other (obesity) is getting worse.

So fast is the rise in morbid obesity that policy morphs swiftly. In the summer of 2010, the UK's influential National Institute for Health and Clinical Excellence aggressively pushed the government to reduce salt and harmful fat content for the whole food industry. It also supported banning TV advertising for fatty foods until nine p.m. to 'protect children,' and encouraged cities to 'restrict planning permission for take-aways and other food retail outlets.' In Ontario, Canada's largest province, with 14 million people, the government announced in June 2009 that it would be expanding access to bariatric surgery by creating a large bariatric network and boosting the number of annual surgeries for XXL-sized individuals in the province to 2,085 a year by 2011–12. That is almost as many as were performed in all of Canada during 2008–9 (2,385), and this number represents a 92 per cent jump between 2004 and 2005. (Bariatric surgery is the surgical fix that limits food intake and caloric absorption. It is clinically indicated only for patients with a BMI over 40, or a BMI over 35 and an additional risk factor such as diabetes.)

After Ontario provided new money for bariatrics, Quebec's health minister chipped in with millions for his province. Surgical needs are hard to predict, but at least surgery is an intervention of proven effectiveness – for some. After surgery, once-obese people generally live longer. We know, for example, that gastric bypass surgery for XXL-sized individuals cuts cancer mortality in half. It also reverses diabetes overnight and stops hypertension and obesity-related arthritis. New surgical techniques have cut down on post-operative bleeding and infection, making this approach ever safer for the morbidly obese.

Those who are one hundred pounds or more overweight – XXXL – constitute the fastest-growing segment of overweight individuals in the United States. More than 7 per cent of American boys and 5 per cent of American girls are XXXL, according to a study published in March 2010 in the *Journal of Pediatrics*. Research has uncovered the fact that in the U.S., the proportion of severely obese adults was 50 per cent higher in 2005 than it had been five years earlier. What happened between 2000 and 2005? Maybe people stopped smoking and took up eating instead. This is not an implausible explanation; America is more obese than most other industrialized nations, but it now boasts relatively low rates of smoking and alcoholism.

Two-thirds of all Americans are already overweight or obese. If the trends of the past three decades are allowed to continue, every single American adult could be overweight approximately forty years from now.[33] This is a theoretical statistical forecast, foretold in a research paper that hit the media with an attention-grabbing press release, and is deliberately provocative.

Whatever the future may hold, the costs of corpulence are crippling health systems today. Roughly 90 per cent of expensive hip and knee replacements – among the most common outpatient surgeries in advanced industrialized countries – are performed on the large to extremely large older populations in Canada, the United States, and Britain. Half a million knee replacements cost the U.S. more than $11 billion in 2005, and the number of such surgeries is growing rapidly due to increased life expectancy and increased rates of obesity.

Childhood obesity rates have nearly quadrupled in the past three decades. The number of children with chronic illnesses is nearly four times the rate it was a generation ago. Amid the cavalcade of data we are presenting, the most significant statistic is the *rate of change:* In 1960, 1.8 per cent of American children and adolescents were reported to have a chronic health condition that limited their activities. By 2004, the rate had risen to 7 per cent, and, these being survey data solicited from parents asked about their child's weight, it was probably higher since parents who are asked these questions generally underplay their child's difficulties. There are knock-on effects. Chronically ill children are by necessity sedentary and, for that reason, put on weight, which means we can anticipate a flood of chronically ill young adults with weight-related illnesses, such as diabetes and heart disease, among other tribulations.

The overall U.S. data (at the time of writing) suggest that 32 per cent of America's children are either overweight or obese.[34] Over thirty years, the percentage of overweight U.S. children and adolescents has tripled: from 5.2 per cent between 1971 and 1974, to 17.3 per cent between 2001 and 2004. Lack of exercise, unhealthy diets, and genetics are most often blamed. But there are many other factors at play. We will look at the litany of assumed causes for the obesity trend lines in the next chapter of this book. Whatever the cause of weight gain for any one individual, childhood obesity matters for long-term health. Fat kids tend to become fat adults, with U.S. adults coming out at 54 per cent overweight or obese according to the latest figures. And fat mothers, as we have seen, bear fatter children. As go mothers' waistlines, so goes the world.

In Canada where we live, the news is grim. There has emerged a category of 'super-obese.' 'We're seeing more severely obese patients and more severity in the severely obese,'[35] Dr Raj Padwal, medical lead of the Capital Health Regional Obesity Program in Edmonton, told the *National Post* in 2008. Our current reality is this: Doctors' offices and weight loss centres have furnished their waiting rooms and diagnostic machines with extrawide, heavily reinforced chairs known as bariatric chairs. Canada's publicly funded health system cannot afford to pay for the special chairs and wheelchairs that are needed by the severely overweight. People are dying on waiting lists in wealthy countries like Canada and the UK because there is grossly insufficient system capacity to perform needed bariatric surgery. Simply put, there is insufficient capacity and there are too few physicians to deal with XXLs – medically, psychologically, surgically, and financially; and this is harming all industrialized countries. The only country that publicly boasts a lack of obesity is North Korea, a totalitarian state; there is no independent verification of that country's dubious obesity data, and, were this unlikely claim true, this would likely be the result of gross malnutrition under the stranglehold of authoritarian communism.

The Global Costs of Obesity

We face a phenomenon of 'globesity.' The World Health Organization has noted that for every four adults in the world who are malnourished, five others are overweight (30 per cent of whom are obese).[36] There are more than one billion overweight people in the world, compared to 800 million who are undernourished. (Paradoxically, the undernourished are often obese. In Western cities, there are few supermarkets in impoverished neighbourhoods, and the ones that do exist carry more processed foods than seasonal fruits and vegetables. Thus the poor get fat but remain undernourished.) Well into the 1960s, even a middle-class, one-income household faced challenges 'putting food on the table.' Now, food is cheap and plentiful for all except the very poorest members of the Western world; the challenge is keeping it off the table and out of our mouths.

Great Britain boasts one of the highest adult obesity rates in the world, and British children are not far behind their parents. The Japanese, who on average live longer than anyone else, are seeing hamburgers, fried chicken, and instant noodles replace the fish, rice, and miso soup that once kept them so slim. Yesterday's media perceptions about 'fit nations' are out the door. In Sweden, obesity rates have doubled in twenty-five years (despite school soda pop bans).[37] Wales reports that fully half of its primary school-aged boys will be obese by 2050.[38] Fifty-two per cent of adults in Spain and almost 28 per cent of Spanish children are either overweight or obese, according to a 2006 study. That puts 2010 World Cup–winning Spain on a par with Britain as one of the largest nations in Europe, even though Spaniards have nurtured a proud reputation and brand of health consciousness, athleticism, and prudent eating. No country, it seems, is immune from the fat epidemic. All industrialized countries are aware of the obesity crisis, but policy makers appear blind to its mounds of complexity and to its dire financial consequences.

You don't have to live in an economically prosperous country to be obese. One of the world's bulkiest populations lives on Nauru, a small island in the central Pacific. Life is mostly sedentary, and the food is fatty. The life expectancy for males is about fifty-five years. Malaysia's health minister, Chua Soi Lek, warned in April 2007 that an epidemic of weight-related illness would hit Malaysia within the next ten years unless ways were found to manage obesity rates. Malaysia is said to have the largest obese population in Southeast Asia. In impoverished Cuba, 30 per cent of men and women are overweight, according to a study done in 2004. The Cuban Communist government supplements the diets of its citizens with baskets of rice, beans, potatoes, bread, eggs, fish, chicken, and a little meat. Cubans also get subsidized meals at work and at school. The government provides one-third of the daily 3,300 calories that each Cuban consumes, yet government-run vegetarian restaurants are apparently nearly empty; starch and pork have greater appeal. (Bizarrely, despite these obvious health and lifestyle concerns, the Cuban health care system, with its high doctor-to-patient ratio, is occasionally held up by academics as an ideal model of health care delivery in some countries – notably Canada, where the opposition Liberal health critic, a physician and professor of medicine, lauded the system in a travel memoir.)

China, too, is struggling to address an obesity epidemic, with more than 25 per cent of its population classified as overweight or obese. Obesity rates in China are part of an economic boom that has brought more wealth to families, so that they spend more money on food. There are now more animal-source foods such as eggs, poultry, beef, and pork in the Chinese diet. Physically demanding occupations are becoming history as more and more people work at sedentary service-sector jobs, drive instead of walk, and spend their leisure time watching TV. In 1989, 63 per cent of households owned a television set; today it would be close to 100 per cent. Chinese public health authorities badly want citizens to eat fruit, vegetables, and high-fibre foods such as soybeans, and to reduce their intake of fat and caloric sweeteners. The government also wants people to exercise – so it tells them to in expensive TV ads. We happen to think that such ads don't work, as we will discuss at length in chapters 3 and 4. If the Chinese don't exercise, the rise in chronic disease could kill up to 80 million people in China over the next decade. Researchers predict a doubling of the problem by 2028 unless something changes.

More than one-third of African women and one-quarter of African men are estimated to be overweight, and the WHO predicts that this will rise to 41 per cent for women and 30 per cent for men in the next ten years.[39] The traditional African diet is heavy in starch, with staple foods like maize meal and white bread. In many African countries, it is not unusual to see people put three spoons of sugar in coffee and tea. Such habits cannot easily be unlearned. That even Africa – a continent synonymous, for many, with hunger and starvation – is experiencing a widespread rise in obesity rates, was a revelation to us. One of the problems is a traditional African belief system that says, 'the larger you are, the more beautiful you are.' Consider these interviews from a BBC documentary in 2006: 'I grew up with low self-esteem and no self-worth due to name calling because of my body structure. To African society, I was just too skinny. I was called names like "bonga fish," "long rat" and other horrible names'; and, 'Being a native of Zimbabwe I can assure you that being chubby is a sure sign of health and wealth in Zimbabwe. With the AIDS epidemic sweeping the country, being chubby is a clear sign that perhaps one is not suffering from the dreaded disease.'[40] In many parts of Africa, however, the definition of beauty is apparently changing, coming closer to the Western ideal.

As we look at nations around the globe, we see that obesity, though common to every region, differs in national character; it differs in its consequences in the two sexes; it differs according to age and personality and socio-economics and genes. It becomes obvious that 'mass market' public health solutions and 'national strategies' to tame obesity will fail.

As the fictional character Philip Von Zweck says in *The Onion*, a satirical online magazine: 'I've heard there are public-service announcements that address the obesity problem, but I don't really see how a commercial is going to make me stop eating. You see, odds are I'm in the kitchen making a sandwich during commercials.'[41]

2 (Nearly) Everything Causes Obesity, and (Almost) Everyone Is Different

From Thin to Fat in One Generation

In the early 1960s, the average American male weighed 168 pounds. That's what heart-throb Cary Grant weighed. Today's male matinee idol, George Clooney, about the same height, normally weighs in between 185 and 195 pounds, though his weight fluctuates. Movie stars readily gain and lose weight for movie roles, so it's hard to pin them down to a steady weight. For the average American woman, weight since the 1960s has shot up from 142 pounds to about 152. Consider that in 1980 only about one-third of Americans were considered overweight and 13 per cent obese. In 1978, Americans ate on average 1,826 calories a day; now it's 2,157. Today it's estimated that over 60 per cent of us in the West are in the overweight category and 25 per cent are obese as defined by BMI levels. Children have been putting on weight at an alarming rate. In 1981 the typical forty-five-year-old Canadian male at 5'8" weighed about 171 pounds compared to 191 by 2008. For females of the same age at 5'4", weight ballooned from 139 pounds to 151 over the same period of time. At ages forty to sixty-nine, the percentage of males and females whose waist circumference placed them at high risk for health problems more than doubled between 1981 and 2009; at ages 20 to 39 years, these percentages more than quadrupled.

The WHO estimates that over one billion people are currently overweight.[42] Over 300 million people fall into the obese category. More than 2.5 million deaths annually are weight-related, and this could rise to 5 million by 2020. The U.S. will be spending 19 per cent of its gross domestic product on health care by 2014, up from 15 per cent in 2003.

Of this, as much as 20 per cent, depending on the calculation, will ulti-mately go toward treating obesity diseases. Yet even with this spend-ing, 'the steady rise in life expectancy during the past two centuries may soon come to an end' as a result of obesity trends, according to a 2005 paper in the *New England Journal of Medicine*.[43] By 2015, more than 1.5 billion people may be overweight, according to the WHO. Marie Ruel of the International Food Policy Research Institute has pointed out that many in the developing world are 'moving from hunger to obesity in a single generation.'[44]

Why We Gain Weight: Many Theories, Basic Facts

Once we stop growing, our intake of energy and our output of energy should balance. If what we take in equals what we put out, our weight stays put. Why, then, does this not automatically happen? *Why* do we gain weight? There are many, many reasons; some are outgrowths of evolving science, and some are based on reasoned speculation. Unde-niably, there are chemical factors that operate at certain times and in certain people to increase input or decrease output. There are inborn genetic factors that favour more build-up or more breakdown of nutri-ents, and these genetic factors may be lying around not doing any-thing until they are aroused from sleep by a stressor (such as divorce, for example); or by a hormone (say, from your thyroid gland); or by a random environmental event such as an elevator installed in your low-rise so that you no longer have to climb stairs every day. Hormo-nal transitions such as pregnancy or menopause, alterations in diet, and changes in activity level due perhaps to illness or to the regular use of a car for commuting to work all may contribute. Psychologi-cal factors play an important role. As we have seen, obesity is often strongly linked to depression, and vice versa. Men and women who are obese have a 55 per cent chance of becoming depressed, and depressed individuals have a similar risk (slightly higher) of becom-ing obese. For reasons we can speculate about but do not know, this association seems to be stronger in the U.S. than in Europe. Certainly in North America, eating comfort foods like pasta and grilled cheese sandwiches soothes emotional pain – a self-treatment commonly resorted to whenever we face anxiety, loneliness, boredom, or anger. 'Stressed spelled backwards is desserts,' psychologists like to say. Oprah Winfrey has said of her famous weight problems: 'I didn't love food – I used food to numb my negative feelings. It didn't matter what the feeling was … no matter how insignificant the discomfort, my first reaction was to reach for something to eat, unaware of how much I was consuming.'[45]

There are ethnic and cultural factors that can promote obesity (traditional foods, celebratory festivals, pride in cookery); there are also socioeconomic factors. In the more developed countries, the poorer you are, the more overweight you tend to be (because inexpensive foods tend to be fatty foods), but this is not the case in countries like China and Malaysia or in South America or sub-Saharan Africa. In these developing countries, the richer you are, the fatter you tend to be, because in these nations, where there is so much poverty, the status symbol is sometimes (but less and less so today) to be able to eat as much as you want. In some Hispanic communities in America, a chubby child may signify that your family is doing well financially. Plump equals healthy, and becoming assimilated means eating fast food. Obesity is a community issue that needs to be understood in context.

As noted in chapter 1, there are specific illnesses that are typically associated with weight gain – hypothyroid conditions, for instance. As we develop better pharmaceuticals for these and other disorders, more and more these very medications may become the actual *cause* of weight gain. They interact with metabolic pathways to make us expand. But this is an individual matter, because drugs have different effects in different people; it depends on your genetics.

For many, obesity can be viewed as an addiction to food. Marlon Brando, who had a family history of alcohol problems, used to say that, unlike most of his family, his addictive poison was food, not alcohol. We now speak about addictions in a broader sense than we used to in the past. We recognize that people can be addicted to sex or to food just as they are to alcohol or drugs. Brain imaging studies have shown that the same areas of the brain that light up when an addictive drug is consumed also light up when food is consumed. Opiate blockers can reduce the craving for narcotics and also the craving for food. Certain kinds of food in particular (sweet or salty or fatty) have a potential for abuse, just like street drugs do. Evolutionary theory says that food craving was an advantage in olden days – it helped survival in times of famine. But this is no longer the case. Food is plentiful now, and the evolutionary advantage has re-emerged as a weapon of self-destruction. Even with a private chef and dietician and psychologist and trainer, Oprah Winfrey struggles with food addiction. You cannot avoid keeping food in the house, as you can with drugs or alcohol or cigarettes. It's always there, forever tempting, and you end up overusing it. Organizing a personal environment that supports weight loss is very hard.

One novel explanation for the obesity epidemic is the reduction in cigarette smoking. We smoke less, so we eat more. We often hear our friends say, 'As soon as I quit smoking, I put on weight.' Other research has suggested that obesity is a social virus; if our friends are fat, we'll be fat. If we associate with the slim, we'll stay slim. Over 12,000 people who had been enrolled in a heart study were followed to see whether weight gain in one person was correlated with weight gain in friends, brothers and sisters, spouses or neighbours. When one sibling became obese, the chance that the other would as well increased by 4 per cent or even 5 per cent if the siblings were of the same sex. When a spouse became obese, the likelihood that the other spouse would follow suit was increased by 3 per cent. Good friends had the highest risk of all. When one became obese, the other had a strong likelihood of becoming obese as well.[46] There was no effect on risk when it was an immediate neighbour who was not also a friend.

The authors of this book are close friends and understand the meaning of friendship, the uniqueness of deep interpersonal relationships. This has helped us contemplate the answers to the question that drove us to write this book. Our purpose was to understand why so many smart political leaders and policy makers have failed to slow down the global obesity epidemic. In debating with each other, and writing (and rewriting upon reflection and further debate), we have learned this much: friendship is a personal, social, and public relationship; preventing and managing weight gain may also be partly social and public, but above all, it is deeply private and intensely personal. As such, controlling obesity eludes the simple and sweeping assumptions so often encountered in public health research and government planning, assumptions that lead to simple models of cause and effect. Furthermore, if managing obesity is such a personal battle, this calls into question the validity of vocal public health campaigns such as: 'pay attention to your five food groups or else!' (To this topic of social marketing, we will return in chapter 3.)

We will long remain co-authors and friends, sharing each other's confidences and personal crises. In life, friendships matter. Friendships serve as incentives to act out certain courses of action or inaction. They also fuel our successes and cushion our failures. But at the same time, we all remain deeply alone in our battles with weight control. This is as science and nature have conspired. Even within intimate personal relationships, none of us fully know the personal anguish that significant others undergo – spouses, parents, even children – when they do battle with weight gain. With our weight struggles, we live and die alone. It is to ourselves that we are accountable. Support from within our network of family and friends helps keep us on track, but no one other than ourselves, certainly not the state, can goad us into action.

According to another recent study, this time in the *Journal of the American Medical Association*, each of us has an individual weight 'set point.'[47] If we eat a little more one day, we may put on some extra weight, but we'll quickly dissipate it and return to our set point. The same applies, unfortunately, when we say 'no' to those tempting cookies. We'll reap a little weight loss benefit the next day, but it won't last. Our bodies will adjust. Why, then, does the set point fail us at some junctures in our lives? Why do we suddenly bulk up or thin down? That's a question to which there are millions of different answers, perhaps a different answer for each of us.

A compelling explanation of the cause of the obesity epidemic highlights that better technology has made prepared food more accessible and relatively cheap. Much-heralded economists, notably Richard Posner and Thomas Philipson, have presented data that show that the growth in obesity is a function of the same technology that created mass-produced meals.[48] Food has become cheaper, and more meals are eaten outside the home. It is easier to stick to a diet when you eat at home, but again, it depends on the person. Many people eat out all the time and stay slim. Some people eat all the no-nos – corn syrup, salty cereal, trans fats – and they still stay slim. On the other hand, some chew on coca leaves, take the Mediterranean diet, faithfully swallow conjugated linoleic acid, and get eight hours of sleep, and they still keep putting on weight.

Chances are that you have a sibling or friend or neighbour or mother-in-law who holds strong opinions as to why so many of us are fat. ('It's all because of TV,' they might say.) They may be right that TV is the culprit as far as they personally are concerned because many people know what their own weak spot is. But their explanation doesn't necessarily hold for you. For you, it may not be TV at all. For you it may be eating ice cream at night when everyone's asleep – a secret indiscretion. Among many conservative-leaning commentators, it is now increasingly the vogue to argue that obesity is the result of people not eating together as a family. Empirically, there is some observational support for this: in 1978, Americans ate 18 per cent of their food outside the

home; in 2006 it was 37 per cent. This has caused concern among prominent conservative-leaning observers such as British physician Anthony
Daniels, who has argued that these circumstances encourage children
to 'graze and forage' rather than eat properly ('Children are like Pooh
Bear, for whom it is always time for a little snack,' he has written in
the *Wall Street Journal*). But this fact doesn't explain why you or your
children may be obese; or why you may eat too many carbohydrates, or
too little protein. Just as important, it is fantasy to expect the fast-paced,
frenetic life of the modern family to return to the Leave-It-to-Beaver
days of regular home-cooked, sit-down meals without interruptions
from the BlackBerry.

There are many, many causes of weight gain and the inability to lose
weight. Some of the causes apply in one case; others apply in other cases. Struggles with weight are individual. There is nothing that works
for everyone or even for a significant minority of people. The results
of most generic weight loss programs are dismal. About 10 per cent of
body weight can be lost during a weight loss program (more than that
is generally not considered safe), but two-thirds of people gain most of
it back within a year, and within five years, 90 to 95 per cent of weight
lost is regained. Why do weight loss programs not work? No one
knows for sure, but public health researchers and health professionals
have very little incentive to say 'I don't know' when investigating the
cause of obesity or its prevention or its treatment. Quite the opposite
– grant funding in the research community is contingent on proving a
hypothesis true, and often, as well, on fitting this hypothesis into a prescribed, politically correct obesity research narrative that assigns blame
to the food industry and that concocts a vegetable soup of fashionable
ideas to address the problem – for example, promoting healthy school
meals or nutritious snacks, banning soda pop in schools, generating
'diversity friendly' urban plans, widening bicycle lanes, or providing
more subsidies for farmers to produce local vegetables, fish, and fruit.
Obesity interventions in public health systems are often designed for
everyone, as if we all can benefit from the same intervention. We want
to challenge this point of view.

Our Public Health Challenge Right Now

Around the world, we're currently taking in vastly more calories than
did our great-grandparents, one-third of whom were probably farmers
still growing their own food. Today in North America, only about 2 per

cent of us are farmers. We are not suggesting a retreat to agrarian society. Even if this were possible, there is no evidence this would return us to a period of healthy weights.

Obesity is the public health challenge of our time. We know that poverty is linked to ill health, but obesity is not just an affliction of the poor. It cuts across most income levels, and it generally defies what economists and public health experts describe as the 'reverse income gradient.' People of almost every racial and cultural group are getting fatter. This applies to men and women of all age groups. Very thin Japanese women, for now, seem to be a curious outlier – but outliers quickly change, as we have seen in the once famously slim French and Spanish. Teens throughout the West in particular are much heavier than a generation ago. Doctors, now ethically and legally obliged in some jurisdictions to openly confront their patients' obesity, are seeing a growing incidence of obesity among children as young as four. The definition of obesity for children is not usually based on body mass index but rather on the percentage by which their weight exceeds that expected for their height. Obesity is an especially serious problem among Native American children, Mexican American children, and African American children. As a parent, you worry every day whether your children will become obese adults and die prematurely of heart problems. You also ask: What kind of life will these children have? They may be teased at school; they may develop Type 2 diabetes (as noted in chapter 1, more and more children are being diagnosed with this historically adult disease) as well as high blood pressure (in kids!), high cholesterol (in kids!), and liver and kidney disease. And of course, the girls may have trouble getting pregnant and may well give birth to high-risk children. The spiralling growth of obesity-related problems needs a strong policy solution.

The paradox is that, as parents pay more and more attention to eating healthy, and as they become 'nutritionally correct,' they (and their children) are getting fatter and fatter and fatter. Our suspicion is that parents are being tricked by what has been called the 'health halo' effect. Because they work so hard at eating naturally processed organic food and avoiding all the 'bad' foods, they forget to look at portions. Since it's presumed to be healthy food, why not eat a lot of it? (This phenomenon is similar to 'risk compensation' in economics: people drive faster on safer, flatter roads.) Why not feed your kids a lot of it? But 'healthy food' contains calories too.

Lisa Dorfman, a registered dietitian and Director of Sports Nutrition at the University of Miami, told the *New York Times* that she treats children who are scared of parent-designated 'bad' foods.[49] 'It's almost a fear of dying, a fear of illness, like a delusional view of foods in general,' she says. 'I see kids whose parents have hypnotized them. I have five-year-olds that speak like 40-year-olds. They can't eat an Oreo cookie without being concerned about trans fats.' Surely this is not the way to get kids to stay trim. There must, we feel, be better ways.

Humility and the Science of Obesity

We must be humble in describing the causes of obesity, since scientific findings change every day. Even BMI, which is how obesity has long been measured, is today having its value questioned. We estimate that the amount of new scientific literature published on the causes of obesity is enough to fill a two-hundred-page book every day. Obesity is the result of a rich combination of factors ranging from highly available, energy-dense food – a late twentieth-century success story traceable to the efficient development of food production technologies, fuelled in part by farm subsidies – to the reduced expenditure of calories due to modern-day conveniences such as microwaves and laptops. Add to that the modern conveniences of lighting, heating, and air conditioning and you realize that our body rhythms are out of touch with the natural cycles that once told us when to eat and when to stop eating. Eating and sleeping and eliminating waste have lost their natural rhythms.

In 2008, each of the factors cited below was identified as a primary environmental driver of obesity in the peer-reviewed public health and nutrition literature (a different combination of all these factors probably applies to each of us):

Car dependency	Every extra hour in a car boosts obesity
'Food apartheid'	Neighbourhoods with supermarkets have less obesity
City planning	Suburbs without jobs, schools, or recreational facilities promote car use
Elevators	Friendly, open stairs promote stair climbing
Suburb design	Curvy, blocked-off streets discourage walking
Portion size	The bigger the portion, the more you eat and drink
Safety and beauty	Safe, attractive parks promote healthy activity and active transport

Fast food saturation	Easy access to fast food promotes a fatty diet
Public transport	Accessible public transport encourages walking
Advertising	Advertisements promoting high-fat, high-sugar foods target kids

If someone were to objectively review the science of obesity, combing the literature carefully, he or she might reasonably conclude that pretty much *everything* about modernity causes obesity: child food allergies, genetics, earlier onset of puberty in girls, excessive consumption of linoleic acid (omega 6), a deficiency in alpha-linolenic acid (omega 3), sleep deprivation, heat, soda pop (including zero-calorie diet pop!).

Yet many of the popular public health solutions above are based on the 'one for all' argument. One person's obesity problem cannot be solved by a policy designed for a statistical majority. To think that it can be is a false generalization that leads to much-hyped 'national strategies' or 'system approaches' to combat obesity – strategies and approaches that do not work. We examine this policy error in depth in chapter 3.

Even intellectual work has been suggested as a cause of obesity![50] Dr Angelo Tremblay measured the spontaneous food intake of fourteen students after each of three tasks. The first task was thoughtful contemplation (that is, doing absolutely nothing). The second was reading and summarizing a written text. The third was completing a series of memory, attention, and vigilance tests on the computer. All three groups of students were then given as much food as they wanted. It was found that those in the latter two groups – the intellectual work groups – consumed over two hundred more calories than the students in the do-nothing group. It seems that just thinking stresses you out, and you eat to compensate.

Theoretical explanations for obesity are widely touted in academic journals, yet there is no gold standard 'randomized control trial' to prove success for *any* of the costly interventions most recommended by public health policy makers. Consider, for example, the idea that a lack of green space fuels obesity – this is speculation. It makes ideological sense if you're an environmentalist, but is it really an important factor for many of us? Think of your obese friends, or someone close to you. Did a lack of park space or a small backyard make them fat? If you know them well enough, you know that something more specific to them caused the sustained weight gain. Energy expenditure can take place on an indoor staircase. Green spaces are great for good city living and family fun, but they are not essential for keeping your weight down, certainly not for most of us.

Because of the wide number of ostensible causes for obesity, it is helpful to broadly categorize them. Understanding the complexity of these causes can help policy makers judge whether various policy ideas would make the slightest bit of difference. Let's start with what's most basic: our genetic make-up as it has evolved over forty thousand years since the Upper Paleolithic period.

Our Genes Make Us Fat

In *The Evolution of Obesity*, the authors turn to Darwin to solve the obesity mystery.[51] Michael Power and Jay Schulkin argue that our big brains are the root cause. Here's their case: As our brains increased in size over time from *Australopithecus afarensis*, who lived 3 million years ago, cranial capacity went from four hundred cubic centimetres (the same as a chimp) to about thirteen hundred cubic centimetres. This change resulted in a lot of energy being required to keep the brain going. And since early humans lived pretty much day to day and hand to mouth, they needed to stockpile food as much as possible, not by squirrelling it away in caves (because we're not squirrels), but by the brilliant trick of storing it in body fat. After all, body fat is rich in energy and rather light in weight. The authors back up their contention by arguing that a gram of fat equals 9.4 kilocalories, compared to 4.3 kilocalories for a gram of protein.

Humans in the Pleistocene would pack on the fat and store it whenever they had a chance, and chances were few and far between because of the unforgiving environment. Those humans whose genetic make-up favoured storing fat were sought after as mates and ended up having the most offspring, so those fat-storing genes got passed on and on until here we are, many millennia later, reaping the advantage of the fat-storing genes. Except that, today, these genes are no longer advantageous. We no longer live in a nutrient-deprived world, and the human body is now exposed to limitless calories in what Power and Schulkin call a 'mismatch paradigm': 'We evolved on the savannahs of Africa. We now live in Candyland.'

Incidentally, not only were our prehistoric ancestors genetically programmed to store fat, but there is also a notion that their limited diet made them healthier. Today some diet books actually want us to go back to caveman diets such as the one described in *The Paleo Diet* by Loren Cordain.[52] That one stresses meats and root vegetables and gets us away from grain-based foods, sugars, and dairy products. Ray Audette, the author of *NeanderThin*, conducted research that led him to adopt a Paleolithic, hunter-gatherer, caveman diet as well.[53] After one month he had lost twenty-five pounds. Audette suggests that modern man should eliminate foods that need human intervention before they are edible. These foods include milk, grains (wheat, corn, rice, oats, barley, and rye), beans, potatoes, alcohol, and sugar. Audette's rule is that if a fruit or vegetable is edible raw without processing, then it is safe to eat. He suggests eating fruits only when they are in season and limiting winter intake of fruits so that the body can burn stored fat. In summary, his advice is to eat meat and fish, fruit, vegetables, nuts, seeds, and berries and to avoid all else. This is fascinating as a matter of personal experimentation, but it does little to solve the obesity problem for the rest of us; this diet won't take hold in poorer neighbourhoods, for example, where fresh fruit is more expensive than bready food and is harder to come by.

Albert Stunkard, an obesity researcher from the University of Pennsylvania, wanted to know how much of the variation in body weight is caused by genes.[54] He and his colleagues recruited 93 pairs of identical twins who were reared apart and 154 pairs of identical twins who were reared together in addition to 218 pairs of fraternal twins who were reared apart and 208 fraternal pairs who were reared together. The identical twins, whose average age was fifty-eight at the time of the study, turned out to have nearly identical BMIs, whether they were reared apart or together; the fraternal twins showed more variance, even when raised together.

No one makes the case strongly that obesity is controlled by *one* gene. Rather, obesity must be the product of subtle interactions among multiple genetic and environmental factors (modern lifestyle and dietary habits leading to over or under expression of specific genes). Depending on the genes you inherit, you may be very much (or not at all) predisposed to get fat when exposed to the modern 'obesogenic environment' (that is, public health speak for a sedentary lifestyle, easy access to processed food, and increased caloric intake). Evolution has better adapted human bodies against weight loss than against weight gain, since for thousands of years our species lived in circumstances where food was scarce. So chances are that relatively few of us have inherited genes that can protect us against putting on more weight than we should. If we continue living in plenty, such genes will be naturally selected and will prosper, but none of us want to wait that long.

Is it genetics that allows some people to eat what they like and not put on weight, while others struggle and still can't get it right? In 1967, when it was still considered appropriate to conduct research on prisoners, a medical researcher, Ethan Sims, recruited Vermont prison inmates and invited them to eat as much as they could. The incentive: if they could gain 25 per cent of their body weight, they would be released from prison early. They all tried, but some just couldn't do it, even though they gorged on 10,000 calories a day.

More recently, Claude Bouchard of Laval University in Quebec and his colleagues studied twelve pairs of identical twins who were all lean to begin with.[55] The twins agreed to remain isolated in a dormitory for the 120 days of the study. After a twenty-day observation period, they were fed an extra 1,000 calories a day, six days a week: a total of 84,000 calories more than they were eating before they entered the study. Each twin of a twosome gained almost exactly the same amount of weight and gained it in the same places as his or her twin. One pair gained the weight in the abdomen, another in the buttocks or thighs. There were important differences among the twin pairs in the amount they gained, from a low of nine-and-a-half pounds to a high of twenty-nine pounds. The average weight gain for the group as a whole was nearly eighteen pounds. The twins who gained the least added more muscle than fat, and those who gained the most added mostly fat. The participants seemed to have inherited a tendency to convert extra calories to either muscle or fat. Since it takes nine times more energy to turn food into muscle than it does to turn it into fat, the twins who put on muscle ended up burning off most of their extra calories.

Scientists have identified several dozen genes that appear to be connected with obesity in humans. There may be as many as two hundred altogether. That means that those who become obese may harbour combinations and permutations of the DNA code of two hundred possibilities – thousands of what geneticists call 'haplotypes,' each unique. Each obese person has a different combination of permutations. So there's no quick fix for obesity, even if gene therapies suddenly became available.

But gene-targeted treatments may ultimately prove critical. For instance, there is a gene variant present in 10 per cent of European and African American populations that is known to be associated to different degrees with obesity. It is located in close physical proximity to the insulin-induced gene 2 (Insig2), which is known to regulate the production of fatty acids and cholesterol. Because of its strategic location, the guess is that the new gene regulates Insig2. The thinking is that this variant must have sprung forth before modern humans left Africa some fifty thousand years ago. The variant was probably harmless until modern times, when some new aspect of the human environment – presumably the wide availability of high-calorie food – interacted with it in such a way as to raise the risk of obesity. Individuals who inherit two copies of the gene variant, one from each parent, have a 22 per cent risk over and above that of the general population of becoming obese. It is not known whether inheriting only one copy raises your risk for weight gain. But the two-copy finding has been replicated in several populations.

Recently, quite a few gene locations have been uncovered that are associated with variations in BMI, but each one accounts for only a very small portion of risk – from 0.05 to 0.24 BMI units only. This suggests that a person needs to be born with many of the two hundred risk genes in order to be susceptible to becoming obese. It has been calculated that carrying twelve such genes increases body weight by six kilograms compared to carrying only one or two.[56] So far, all of the genetic sites that have been discovered definitively explain only about 1 per cent of the genetic variation in any population. Most of the genetic sites until now have been found in European populations; other populations have been less studied. A large amount of genetic variation that controls obesity, therefore, is still awaiting discovery. The fuller identification of genes controlling satiety (the feeling of fullness) and energy expenditure and adipogenesis (the growth of fat cells) will allow for the possibility of specific drug development and individualized cures.

A story from Israel points to another possible genetic lead. The body is composed of fat mass, lean mass, and bone mass. Lean mass is important because it dwindles with age, and understanding it better could help resolve some of the paradoxes of weight and health. Therefore, instead of looking at genes that influence fat, scientists from Tel Aviv University looked for new gene variants that affect lean body mass.[57] Finding genes would, they hoped, lead to the prevention and treatment of obesity as well as to the prevention and treatment of the complications of weight, such as diabetes and cardiovascular problems. Personalized medicine has already paid off for Type 2 diabetes. A therapy tailored to an individual's genes allowed hundreds of diabetes sufferers in Britain to switch from insulin injections to cheaper, more effective drugs after a simple test showed that they had a particular genetic form of diabetes. The test, which is available through the UK's National Health Service (NHS), could end up benefiting up to twenty thousand individuals and saving the NHS at least £30,000 over each patient's lifetime. A second genetic test waiting in the wings could help identify another thirty thousand people with a milder form of diabetes.

So genes contribute to obesity in many ways by affecting appetite, satiety (fullness), metabolism (the way food is digested), food cravings, body fat distribution, and the psychological tendency to use eating as a way to cope with stress. The strength of the genetic influence on weight disorders varies significantly from person to person. Research suggests that for some overweight people, genes account for just 25 per cent of the predisposition to be overweight, whereas for others, the genetic influence may be as high as 70 to 80 per cent. No one knows how big a role genes play in your weight; there are no tools to measure it, but you can assume that if several people in your close family have big bellies, there must be a genetic influence at work. That doesn't mean that cutting down on calories and exercising more often won't be effective for you. It will. But the *way* you cut down and the *way* you exercise needs to rely on your relative strengths and not on your relative weaknesses. If there's something amiss with the message from our brain that tells us we are full and can stop eating, bike lanes or 'green space' in local parks won't help us, as we explain throughout this book. We'll go biking and then eat twice as much when we return. If our problem is resisting high-fat, high-sugar foods, then one-on-one strategies might work – a buddy, a higher purpose, and ten steps. Perhaps in the future, but in the very faraway future, a gene chip will tell us where our weak spots are and we'll automatically know how to address the problem.

An important breakthrough in understanding the influence of genes on people's weight was the discovery in 1994 of the obese, or ob, gene.[58] This gene directs the production of leptin, a hormone secreted by fatty tissue that acts on the brain and influences a person's appetite and metabolism. A gene was also discovered that governs the production of leptin receptors in the brain. Some scientists think that the role of leptin is to help prevent starvation by regulating a person's appetite, emotional desire for food, and metabolism. When a person's fat stores drop below the level needed for survival, leptin levels also plummet. In response, appetite and the desire for food increase and metabolism decreases, leading to an increase in fat storage. The added fat causes the leptin level to rise again. Rising leptin then leads to a decrease in appetite and emotional desire for food and to an increase in metabolism, until the set point we referred to earlier is regained.

Much of what is known about leptin comes from scientific experiments with mice that lack an ob gene and therefore produce no leptin. These mice are extremely obese, but they slim down when given leptin injections. You might think, then, that obese people would show a leptin deficiency, but most do not. Most have high leptin levels. Why so?

Some of us may be overweight because we are insensitive to leptin, in much the same way that people with Type 2 diabetes are insensitive to insulin. In other words, despite a high leptin level, the appetite and desire for food remain high, and metabolism remains low. This is an area of intense research, with no consensus, but one conclusion is self-evident: not all obese people are leptin-insensitive. It is one factor among many that leads to weight gain in some people.

There are many other proteins that help regulate appetite, energy metabolism, and body weight, and this is leading to the development of new drugs for the control of obesity – drugs that are currently undergoing trials for effectiveness and safety. Of particular relevance, the study of leptin and its cousins has shown us that the influence of genes on obesity isn't a one-way street: the internal environment acts on genes (turning them on and off) as much as the other way around. Genes are master switches, but they lie dormant unless something turns them on. Eating a high-fat diet sometimes promotes leptin resistance, though researchers don't yet understand how. And the more obese a person is, the more leptin-insensitive he or she often becomes. The reverse is probably also true – that eating a low-fat diet and losing weight increases a person's leptin sensitivity.

Genetics research has led to a number of immediate benefits. In a study involving 133 overweight women, those with a genetic predisposition to benefit from a low-carbohydrate diet lost two-and-a-half times as much weight as those on the same diet without that particular predisposition.[59] Similarly, women with a genetic make-up that favoured a low-fat diet lost substantially more weight than women without low-fat genes who tried to curb fat calories. Determining a person's genetic predisposition is a new tool to help us decide what diet to go on.

Ethnic and Racial Factors

Though the prevalence of insulin resistance and obesity-related diabetes has increased in the past decades at an alarming rate in all Western countries, studies conducted in diverse populations suggest that some ethnic groups, such as Hispanics and Southeast Asians, may have a particular genetic predisposition to develop obesity-related diabetes. What perhaps once led to the successful evolution of specific ethnic groups may now have become a distinct disadvantage. The environment has changed, and a different set of genes is needed to make the most of it. Traditions, customs, and attitudes shared by ethnic communities contribute as much as genes. Social pressures combine with physical make-up to determine weight.

Environmental Factors

Many researchers think that environmental factors bear the main responsibility for the dramatic increase in obesity in recent years across the West. The prevalence of obesity among adults in the United States has been rising since the 1970s.[60] It soared from 15 per cent in 1980 to 23 per cent in 1994, reaching 26 per cent in 2000, according to national surveys by the U.S. Centers for Disease Control and Prevention. Genes alone cannot possibly explain such a rapid rise, though remember, genes lie dormant until awakened. Something in the environment may have woken them up. The rise in BMI appears to cut across all major demographic groups. Middle Eastern countries report that obesity affects 40 per cent of the population, affecting more women than men. Data from all parts of the world reflect the same worrying trends.

One CDC survey for 1991–8 found little change in Americans' relative physical activity.[61] The percentage of people who admitted to being sedentary held steady at about 30 per cent. And the proportion who said they exercised regularly remained just over 40 per cent. If these reports are accurate, a good explanation for the increase in BMI is that people are simply eating more than they were a decade ago. Contrary to what many people think, we are not eating more high-fat foods – research shows that the fat content of our diet has actually gone down in the past twenty-five years. But many low-fat foods are very high in calories because they contain large amounts of sugar to improve their taste. Many 'low fat' foods are actually higher in calories than foods that are considered highly caloric. Everyday life in North America is full of high-calorie temptations at practically every corner and every shopping centre: ice cream stands, cookie shops, and fast-food restaurants of every ethnic flavour. Enormous servings of food and drink are commonplace, not only in restaurants but also in movie theatres and sports stadiums. A single super-sized meal may contain 1,500 to 2,000 calories – all the calories that most of us need for an entire day. It is generally believed among dieticians that an obese dieter must cut 3,500 calories a day to lose a pound – a crude calculation to be sure. But if true, it would mean that someone who eats a super-size meal a day and is fully sedentary will gain a pound or more every day. (Since everyone's body is different, nutrition experts have recently been re-examining the 3,500-calorie rule.)

In addition, as people work longer hours and balance the increasingly challenging demands of job and family, they cope with the time crunch by eating prepared foods, ordering takeout, or eating in restaurants. As many working mothers asked us, 'Does anyone cook anymore?' Reliance on prepared foods often means meals that are larger and higher in calories than a typical meal would be if cooked at home. Americans are consuming more and more calories in the form of sodas and other sweetened drinks sold in ever-larger containers. Some researchers think that the very act of eating irregularly, frequently, and on the run may be contributing to obesity. New neurological evidence indicates that the brain's biological clock – the natural pacemaker that controls numerous other daily rhythms in our bodies – may also help regulate hunger and fullness. Inner signals are supposed to keep our weight steady. They should prompt us to eat when our body fat falls below a certain level or when we need more body fat (during pregnancy, for example), and they should tell us when we've had enough and when it's time to stop eating. Close connections between the brain's appetite centre and its timing centre suggest that hunger and fullness are controlled by time cues. Irregular eating patterns can disrupt these cues.

The Role of Technology

It has been suggested that technology and economically related factors also conspire to make some people fat. Researchers such as Darius Lakdawalla, Tomas Philipson, and David Cutler argue that sedentary jobs and the relatively low cost of food thanks to farming innovations have made us eat more and move less.[62] In other words, food consumption, like everything else, responds to the laws of supply and demand; the lower the relative price of food, the more we consume. One estimate is that 40 per cent of the recent increase in weight may be due to lower food prices. Health economist Eric Finkelstein makes the case that between 1983 and 2005, the real cost of fats and oils declined by 16 per cent; for sugar-laden soft drinks, the decline was 20 per cent.[63] As Finkelstein notes: 'For most people a cold coke used to be a treat reserved for special occasions.' Nowadays, everyone's refrigerator is filled with soft drinks, which account for 7 per cent of all calories consumed in America. American farmers have become skilled at producing (subsidized) corn in massive quantities, making it possible for a Big Mac, fries, and a soft drink to cost just five dollars. The average eat-in restaurant charges that much or more for a fresh salad.

Combine that with lower rates of physical activity, and weight gain is inevitable. Since the 1980s, the number of calories sweated out by adults and children has not changed much while the amount of calories consumed has gone up. Between the mid-1970s and the mid-1990s, men increased their caloric intake by about 268 calories per day (from 2,080 to 2,347); for women, it was 143 calories per day (from 1,515 to 1,658). What accounts for the increase?

It's impossible to answer this question with certainty. As noted, in the 1960s, people cooked their own meals and ate at home more often. Since then there has been a big change in where and how we eat our meals. Technology has led to vacuum-packed foods, food preservatives, deep freezing, artificial flavours, and a slew of microwavable prepackaged foods.

Two other trends over the past several decades have been strongly implicated in the rise in obesity: the decline in smoking that we've already mentioned, and the increasing numbers of women in the labour force. Shin-Yi Chou, Michael Grossman, and Henry Saffer combined the CDC's Behavioral Risk Factor Surveillance System (BRFSS) data with several state-level indicators to examine the impact of increased food consumption away from home and the reduction in smoking, as well as other factors.[64] They found that the more restaurants in a given area, the more weight goes up. Also, the more the price of cigarettes goes up, the more weight goes up. In other words, the more you eat out and the less you smoke, the fatter you get.

Patricia Anderson, Kristin Butcher, and Phillip Levine used matched mother–child data from the National Longitudinal Survey of Youth (NLSY) to investigate how a mother's employment status influences the likelihood that her child will be overweight; they found, as they expected, that when a mother works away from home, her child puts on weight.[65] Instead of small, healthy, home-cooked meals, the child is exposed to pre-packaged, calorie-filled snacks. This politically incorrect finding is not what working moms want to hear: it reinforces the guilt that many of them feel for staying in the workforce and being away from their kids.

What else is making us fat? Many culprits have been cited in the academic press. These include:

1. Corporations produce and promote cheap fast food to please their shareholders.
2. Low funding levels for education mean we don't teach children how to stay healthy.
3. Friends encourage us to eat. They consider it an insult when you leave food on your plate.
4. Cities make us fat since there are no parks, and city logistics make us drive everywhere.
5. Changing family and social patterns make us fat. We socialize around food and TV.
6. Our brains make us fat – they're wired in a way that makes us want to store fat.
7. TV and computers make us fat because they are fun activities that are sedentary.
8. Our addiction to food makes us fat; it's easy to want more when it tastes so good.

Psychological Factors

We all know how our own psychological needs lead to weight gain. One study done by the Scottish Association for Mental Health (SAMH) found that people with mental health problems were four times more likely to be obese than those without. Peter Rice, Chairman of Royal College of Psychiatrists Scotland, said: 'This important survey by SAMH shows the importance of mental health issues in Scotland's health challenges.'[66]

As with most chronic conditions, obesity is very often accompanied by mental health problems. Several studies have shown an association between depressive symptoms and high body mass index. A BMI above 30 among women has been linked to a nearly 50 per cent increase in the lifetime prevalence of depressive disorders. In men, it's abdominal obesity and a high waist-to-hip ratio that correlates with depressive symptoms. Obesity and depression seem to be strongly associated – though oddly, not in everyone. The results of a study sampling 43,534 individuals aged eighteen to ninety (the Continuous Survey of Living Conditions) suggests a U-curve such that very underweight and very overweight individuals are more likely to be depressed than are normal-weight individuals.[67] The neurotransmitters serotonin and norepinephrine are involved in the regulation of both mood and weight, and these are the very transmitters that are targeted by antidepressant drugs. As they relieve depression, antidepressants also induce weight gain so that a vicious cycle ensues: people who are really depressed over their weight are treated with chemical agents that increase their weight even further. At the same time, drugs that are used for weight loss, such as silbutramine and rimonabant, tend to induce depression and have even been accused of provoking suicidal thoughts in some people.

Counter-intuitive as this might seem, weight loss itself can carry a downside for your mental health. It has been reported that suicide occurs with greater than normal frequency not only among those who have lost weight as a result of weight loss medication, but also among those who have lost weight secondarily to lifestyle change. Being heavy can serve a rational purpose for many – perhaps to fend off the opposite sex and avoid unwanted attention. Without that protective barrier, some people feel lost and vulnerable. In other words, losing weight may provoke depression in some people. It is clear that obesity cannot be treated in isolation and must, in many if not all people, be coupled with tackling underlying mental health challenges. Some obese people benefit from cognitive behavioural interventions (CBTs) that target eating habits, dietary choices, or depressive ruminations and self-defeating attitudes. CBT has been found to improve self-reported mental health among some obese people and also to lower their weight. But the initial weight loss doesn't last. People need to be induced to continue lifestyle changes indefinitely, long after the end of CBT.

Weight and mood are definitely connected, but in complex and highly individual ways. Though many factors lead to depression, dietary patterns in the Western world are unquestionably an important part of the mix. There are some data connecting fish consumption with lower population risks of depression and suicide.[68] Also, some studies of depressed patients show an association between low cholesterol and major depression, with recovery linked to an increase in total cholesterol. On the face of it, these findings challenge the vast array of mass public health programs across the United States, Canada, and Europe aimed at lowering cholesterol. Stopping the use of lipid-lowering drugs altogether has even been proposed. Clearly, the issue is complex and at times loaded with contradictions. Any meaningful treatment has to be individualized.

Feeding control, the mechanism that tells us when we are hungry and when we are full, differs among all humans. Satiety, or fullness, is set at different levels, probably a genetic inborn trait. But the foods we eat tend to result in different levels of satiety. For instance, Satiety Index scores (how much a food satisfies hunger) reflect the total amount of fullness produced by set portions of test foods over a set time period.[69] Croissants turn out to be only half as satisfying as white bread (the standard) for most people. Boiled potatoes (but not French fries) are more than three times as satisfying as white bread. A food's chemical composition is one factor that determines how it ranks on the Satiety Index. Beans and lentils contain anti-nutrients, which delay their absorption so that they make most people feel full for long periods of time. In general, the more fibre, protein, and water a food contains, the longer it will give the feeling of fullness (though people differ). Another factor that makes a food satisfying is its sheer bulk. Popcorn is an example. It's the size, bulk, and blandness of potatoes that may account for their high Satiety Index. As a group, fruits rank near the top, with a Satiety Index 1.7 times higher than white bread. Fatty foods, perhaps surprisingly, are not usually satisfying. The reason is that fat, once absorbed, gets stored for a rainy day; it is not broken down for immediate use. That means that when you eat fat, there is no signalling to the brain – as there is with carbohydrates – that enough fuel has been taken in.

Energy efficiency, whereby we turn the energy contained in food into immediate fuels instead of accumulating it as fat, differs among individuals. When we have a fever, our fat stores are converted into heat. That is partly why we lose weight during illness. Calories are used in involuntary movement as well as in heat generation, growth, inflammatory processes, tissue restoration, and metabolism. Many calories are needed for movement.

The process of adipogenesis, or the formation of specialized fat cells, also differs among people. It has always been known that fat cells develop in many different sites scattered throughout the body, generally in the areas of loose tissue between muscle and skin layers. But fat deposits also form around the heart, kidneys, and other internal organs. Recently, stem cell studies have shed light on cell development. Thus far, most scientific work in this area has been carried out on white fat tissue, but mammals, including humans, have a second type of fat cells called brown fat, which dissipates energy instead of storing it. Brown fat produces heat and is therefore important in cold weather; by expending energy it also protects against obesity. So the *kind* of fat you have matters, and *where* it is matters. As mentioned earlier, many adult males have fat, or 'spare tires,' around the abdomen, which predisposes them to diabetes and heart problems; whereas women usually accumulate their fat under the skin, mainly in the thighs and buttocks. The female distribution is less likely to lead to illness. Several key molecules that regulate adipogenesis have been discovered, and a reasonable working model of the network of interactions among these many factors is already known. But much, much more is still unknown. There remain, for instance, important questions about how cells know when to turn into either brown fat or white fat.

The gradual expansion of knowledge about these types of processes is leading toward a better biological understanding of how body weight is regulated. Knowing more about these chains of events is bound to lead to new methods of obesity control. Some people will benefit from one method and some from another, depending on their genetic make-up and the environment in which they live.

Biology is only part of the larger issue of obesity. We need to better understand how social relationships influence food and eating patterns. Immigrants new to the food of their adoptive countries are especially vulnerable to obesity. It has been found, for instance, that, by two years, children of immigrant mothers who do not speak the language of the new country already have higher BMI scores than their peers. Is it breastfeeding practices or dietary intake or feeding habits or physical activity patterns that affect the energy balance of these preschool children? How does the fact that their mother doesn't speak the language of the majority make this happen?

We need to better understand how different groups of individuals interact with their environments in ways that make them eat more and move less. Does, for example, living close to a public community centre inspire recent immigrants from India to venture outside more frequently and partake in physical sports? Sleep specialists have important insights, too. There is some evidence that long sleeps decrease body fat. Children who engage in physical activity sleep more at night than children who tend to watch TV. Not sleeping at night means you're up and tempted to snack. Sleep duration is a potentially adjustable factor that could be important to consider in the prevention and treatment of obesity, especially in childhood. Sleep deprivation is of great concern in the United States, where the latest 2010 data from the National Health Interview Survey show that three in ten adults average six hours of sleep or fewer per night.[70]

From a psychological perspective, individual motivations and particular interests are crucial. By early adolescence, our own interests have already been determined, and these vary widely, from sports, to cooking, to math, to music, to gardening, to reading, to travel. This variety is important to consider when developing intervention programs: What do individuals consider the most enjoyable? What activities are they most likely to commit to? This is why personalized weight loss options, if we can find approaches to supporting and sustaining them, hold so much promise.

An example: For girls who like to read, a new series of books, intended for nine- to thirteen-year-olds, is challenging thin-is-perfect stereotypes, which have been embedded in our culture in girls as young as three. The series Beacon Street Girls, written under the pseudonym Annie Bryant, focuses on many issues, including weight loss. At the annual scientific conference of the Obesity Society in 2009, researchers from the Duke Medical School reported findings on the effects of *Lake Rescue*, a Beacon Street book that focuses on the struggles of an overweight girl named Chelsea Briggs.[71] This is a quote from Chelsea Briggs:

> That's my new goal for this year, believe it or not – to SWEAT more often! That's right. Before I went to Lake Rescue (see Beacon Street Girls book #6 for my story!), I was totally fine just chillin' on the couch eating potato chips and watching TV. Now, after seeing where that kind of lifestyle leads (read: out of breath and out of shape!), I took matters into my own hands. Now, I think every day about how to make it my healthiest day EVER. That doesn't mean working out at the gym for three hours or counting calories. It just means making small choices like taking the stairs instead of the elevator or choosing an apple instead of a candy bar at lunch. Little decisions like that add up to a HEALTHIER lifestyle.

Thirty-one girls were given a copy of 'Lake Rescue'; thirty-three others received a 2006 Beacon Street book, *Charlotte in Paris*, that carries a positive message of self-esteem but doesn't focus on weight or healthful eating. After six months, the girls who read *Lake Rescue* – and many read it more than once – posted a decline in average BMI scores of 0.71;

those who didn't read the book showed an average increase of 0.05. Over time, if this change could be replicated with an entire repertoire of similar books, this difference could emerge as a significant weight management intervention for girls who enjoy reading.

Adults differ markedly in what they consider enjoyable, too. Some busy executives enjoy using a treadmill desk. With a laptop and a phone headset, executives can go all day at a leisurely 1.4 miles an hour. The 'work walker' can burn an estimated 100 to 130 calories an hour at speeds slower than two miles an hour, Mayo Clinic research shows.[72] The treadmill desk is one option among many that the busy professional might choose to commit to in consultation with his or her health professional.

Finding something fun to do to combat weight gain fights obesity head on. It substitutes a healthy pleasure for the unhealthier pleasure of eating sinful but tasty foods. When fats and sugars are consumed in binges, excessive dopamine is released (as happens when you take cocaine); this in turn causes compensatory changes that may be as profound as those caused by drugs of abuse. It is possible that animals that were most eager to seek out the food they needed for survival were the ones who, in fact, survived; that may be the basis for our drug addiction problems today. We have evolved to be avidly on the hunt for that dopamine rush. The resulting weakness of the will is known in Spanish as *abulia*, which is a cruel trick that nature has bequeathed us. This suggests the need for individualized approaches to obesity intervention, akin to those for drug addiction. Public health policy gave up long ago on scary-sounding anti-drug videos with names such as *Reefer Madness*.[73] Almost everyone in marijuana addictions research now recognizes that money must be spent on individualized interventions. Interventions to successfully contain heroin addiction, for instance, are varied; so should be those for food addiction.

Here is what we know about cravings, motivation, and willpower: the amalgam of psychological determinants of obesity is far more complex than that for smoking or drinking. Consider that even with all the professed determination, public scrutiny, and financial resources at her disposal, billionaire Oprah Winfrey suffers intensely with her weight. If she can't manage her weight successfully over the long term, who can? She once recalled the moment that she realized she had to start losing weight. It was at a World Heavyweight bout in Las Vegas – when it hit her that she weighed more than the winner!

President Obama, the 'nudger-in-chief' when it comes to urging children to step away from video games and cut down on junk food ('Finally, a thin president,' blared a headline in the *New York Times* shortly after his election), may think that regulating junk food and TV games is the right solution to the obesity epidemic. But one of his chief advisers, Cass Sunstein, with whom Obama worked closely at the University of Chicago, champions behavioural economics, the economic school of thought that values incentives over penalties. And incentives work best when they are tailored to individual desires and predilections – a topic to which we return in chapter 3.

Changing Public Health Strategies

As we will document in our policy chapters, chapters 3 and 4, public health strategies that are attractive in carefully controlled experimental situations, or on white boards in bureaucrats' offices, are futile in the real-life public health context, in which complex physiological and environmental factors seem to overpower individuals' abilities to control their unique weight challenges. At this period of intense scientific debate about obesity, anyone who professes to know the scientific or clinical 'solution' to obesity is either a faker or naive to the problem's great unknowns. No single thesis enjoys clinical or expert consensus; that said, the four bromides we hear most often are likely to be substantially correct.

Bromide One: 'The problem with obesity stems from people not eating regular square meals.' Certainly, there's probably a correlation between people who eat just three 'squares' a day (with all food groups properly represented) and better health. (Those sentenced to controlled environments – that is, long prison terms – tend to lose significant weight. As noted earlier, one study that tried to fatten up prisoners failed.) Bromide Two: 'Overeating is an addiction.' True again. Tasty food (sugar, salt, and fat, according to David Kessler's *The End of Overeating*) hits on the dopamine or 'pleasure' receptor (the 'D2 dopamine receptor'), resulting in a 'high' much like that of other addictive substances, like cocaine or heroin.[74] More dopamine release generates a hard-wired compulsion to overeat. (Some studies have shown that the obese have fewer dopamine receptors in their brains than lean people.) Bromide Three: 'Eat what you will: just exercise, stupid.' Yes, movement burns off calories. Bromide Four: 'Overeating is a lack of self-control.' It's hard to argue with any of this. It's the successful journey from fat to fit – one individual at a time – that eludes policy makers.

To steal the words of the rock band Buffalo Springfield: 'Nobody's right if everybody's wrong.' Science today understands the metabolism of obesity, insofar as we know what keeps calorie accumulation at bay: more output, less intake. For at least half a century, health agencies and governments (and parents) around the world have been warning about the dangers of obesity, perhaps not as loudly as they could have, but now we all see how obesity-related illnesses have converged in an ugly perfect storm – diabetes, depression, heart disease, and hypertension all are on the increase.

Advances in the science of genetics, in-depth understanding of cultural traditions, appreciation of the impact of neighbourhoods and peer pressure, and exploration of psychological factors will, together, lead to an era of personalized approaches to obesity prevention and treatment. The response of each individual to diet and other environmental factors will vary considerably, depending on individual weight control mechanisms. Future dietary and pharmacological control of obesity will have to take into account each individual's unique response set. Individuals do not respond in the same ways to the same treatments. When taking identical doses of the same drug, some people fare well while others find themselves poisoned. Six to seven per cent of all hospital admissions in the United States are a result of adverse reactions to otherwise innocuous drugs.[75] In that country alone, roughly one hundred thousand deaths a year result from this. There is a wealth of evidence that the individual differences that lead to these deaths are caused by hereditary variations in genes that encode the enzymes responsible for transporting, metabolizing, and excreting these drugs. Statins, for instance, are prescribed to reduce low-density lipoprotein (LDL) cholesterol, but the responses to them are highly variable. Variation in the genes involved in lipoprotein metabolism influences the individual efficacy of statins.

Individuals and particular subpopulations march to different drummers when responding to weight loss activities, and there is no way yet to know in advance who will do better with what regimen. Success, we strongly feel, will depend on the availability of choice – on allowing people to choose what they think will work for them.

Imagine, then, if we developed a policy regimen under which individuals and their families could *choose* a subsidized weight management opportunity from among thousands available. Individuals could commit (perhaps through a personal pledge to their family doctor) to participate in a dance class, or a gardening class (if you grow vegetables, you will be more likely to consume them), or even a study to measure the impact of a new anti-obesity intervention. The key would be to offer real choice among as many options as possible.

Here's a fundamental example of the importance of customized, individually tailored public policy: men and women differ in fat distribution, with women having considerably more of their weight in fat; this difference becomes even more accentuated after menopause. In addition, a recent imaging study published in *Proceedings of the National Academy Science USA* shows that men are better able than women to suppress hunger, to inhibit the brain activation elicited by food.[76] This strongly suggests that men and women react very differently to obesity interventions and that any measure of success will differ between the two sexes. That being so, it follows that measures of success will differ even more greatly among individuals.

Individuality and Paradox

Just one more colourful irony and telling complexity to add to the mystery of obesity is this: dark chocolate and other cocoa-rich foods actually lower blood pressure. Cocoa is rich in a type of antioxidant that lowers blood pressure for some people. Researchers estimate that in certain populations, the blood pressure–lowering effect associated with cocoa could potentially reduce the risk of stroke by about 20 per cent, coronary heart disease by 10 per cent, and death from all causes by 8 per cent.[77] They say those effects are similar to using a beta blocker or an ACE inhibitor (a standard treatment for high blood pressure).

Another unexpected finding: a breakfast of ham and cheese with whole-grain bread and a low-fat spread may lead to better weight control than the less fatty cereal breakfasts that most North American children eat. Sugary foods, such as cornflakes with two spoonfuls of sugar, or waffles and maple syrup, have a high glycemic load (this refers to the rate of release of carbohydrates into the blood stream) and therefore lead to low blood sugar by late morning. Slow glucose release (following a protein meal like ham and cheese) helps curb obesity because there's no midmorning sugar dip and, therefore, no urge to snack. Many Israelis who commonly eat heavy breakfasts may have it right.

Other paradoxes abound: heavier patients who come to the emergency room with clogged arteries have a lower death rate than those who are leaner. This may not be as odd as it looks. It can probably be explained by the fact that arteries clog faster in overweight individuals so that they are comparatively younger when they come to ER and, therefore (because of their younger age), receive relatively more aggressive treatment, and that saves lives. And another paradox: normal-weight women who drink light to moderate amounts of alcohol appear to gain less weight and have less risk for overweight and obesity than non-drinkers, according to the results of a large study reported in *Archives of Internal Medicine*.[78]

Of course, there is good fat and bad fat. Saturated fats are bad for many people. That includes the fat from beef, chicken, pork, and lamb. Also bad are cream, butter, cheese, and milk (except when skimmed). Also, palm oil and coconut. Fish oils and non-animal fats (avocado, nuts, olives and seeds, but not palm oil and coconut) are good fat for many people. A Mediterranean-style diet high in olive oil and other fish and vegetable fats prevents repeat heart attacks just as well as the American Heart Association's recommended low-fat diet. But consider that Mediterranean people are of a specific genetic stock. Maybe Mediterranean-style food is only good for Mediterranean people. Over time, humans and the foods they eat adapt to each other. It's when adaptation is interfered with, when we start eating food to which our bodies are not accustomed (and a lot of it), that troubles come. As Shakespeare said: 'They are sick that surfeit with too much, as they that starve with nothing.'

The largest study ever to ask the question, 'Does a low-fat diet lower the risk of cancer or heart disease?' found that diet has *no effect*. What about drugs? Drugs that lower fat are not always safe and are not always effective over the long term. What about exercise? Generic exercise programs should, theoretically, work for everyone, but they don't, because carrying extra weight is often associated with osteoarthritis and fibromyalgia – joint and muscle pain – which makes exercise very difficult and potentially harmful for some. Obesity is also associated with digestive problems, heartburn, and gall bladder disease, which can all interfere with the ability to exercise. Exercise programs, to work, need to be highly individualized.

A recent study of four popular diets in eight hundred overweight adults found that after two years, every diet group had lost – and regained – about the same amount of weight, regardless of what diet had been assigned. Participants lost an average of thirteen pounds at six months and maintained about nine pounds of weight loss at the two-year mark. Fifteen per cent of dieters had lost more than 10 per cent of their weight by the end of the study. Attendance at counselling (also offered) did not seem to matter. Some people lost large amounts of weight even though they did not attend many counselling sessions. The researcher, Frank Sacks, said: 'We had some people losing 50 pounds and some people gaining five pounds. That's what we don't have a clue about.'[79] What makes some people stick to diets and others not? Is the timing wrong? Is the incentive insufficient? We think it is something about the fit between the person and the diet. In a word: *matching*.

Personalized treatments can be pharmacological or psychological or surgical. Can some of us be taught to feel full though we haven't eaten much? Can some of us be taught to embrace stress-relieving techniques that do not involve food? Can some of us be taught new habits that expend more energy? We already know that certain groups of people (the elderly and those with hypertension, for instance) do not respond well to the surgical procedures that are available for excess weight. We now have to better delineate which procedure, which drug, which motivational message, works best for which individuals. Our task in the rest of this book is to offer a policy solution that will allow health professionals and their patients, working together, to make this happen.

3 One-Size-Fits-Nobody

Distinctiveness and Parental Angst

We've introduced the costs of obesity, and we've talked about many of its complex, interconnected causes (known and unknown). What public health policies have been tried? What has worked? What has failed? We explore the answers to these questions here – but our focus, as before, is on trying to understand weight loss and weight management success for individuals.

One of the tenets of the Western world, and one on a rapid climb, is distinctiveness and individuality. Never before have we invested so much in diversity, in exceptionality, in recognizing that each of us brings special talents and treasures to the world. School curricula, for instance, are 'made to measure' – designed so that education can be matched to every child's unique needs. We're all 'helicopter parents' now; no matter our economic circumstances, we hover over our children to ensure that caring, loving teachers nurture their special creative requirements. We give our children unique names so that they will stand out from the crowd; we carefully pick their schools; we interview their teachers and camp counsellors. It is rare these days to hear anyone saying, 'All kids need the same 3 Rs.' Teachers and parents agree that different children need different curricula.

Yet the march of distinctiveness hasn't penetrated the inner sanctum of the public health bureaucracy, whose job it is to keep us healthy. This, even though concern over their children's weight has reached par with, or exceeded, parental concerns about the quality of their children's education. Of great interest to middle-school parents throughout the West is how far schools accommodate 'healthy living choices' in cafeterias – for example, whether they ban the sale of soda pop. They petition the government to provide funding to public schools so that fresh fruits and vegetables and low-fat milk are freely available at school lunches. They want fast food and soft drink concessions eliminated from public schools, even if it means using federal tax dollars to compensate schools for revenues lost. They want a national network of summer camps that emphasize good nutrition and exercise. They want high-fat, high-sugar food advertising on media watched by children prohibited. Parents are hyperconcerned by the obesity epidemic.

The Failure of a One-Size-Fits-All Approach

What has been the policy response to the epidemic? First, not everyone buys the view that obesity is an 'epidemic.' That illness metaphor implies a spreading contagion. Nor does everyone agree that obesity is an illness at all – many in public health and other disciplines argue that traditional biological medicine has taken over social ills such as obesity, smoking, and alcohol and drug use and 'biologized' them. Be that as it may, there is an impressive biological basis to weight gain, which we have outlined in chapters 1 and 2. The contagion issue is a new perception, referred to earlier, made popular by a 2008 *New England of Journal of Medicine* paper showing that associating with people who are overweight can increase one's own risk of gaining weight.[80]

Public health bureaucrats have responded by throwing large sums of money at 'bully pulpit' policies that advise people to 'eat right and exercise.' These banal bulk messages have been completely ineffective in bringing down the rates of obesity. To understand why, it is instructive to begin with a review of Schools of Public Health, which graduate the students who go on to craft obesity policy. Those schools graduate advocacy coordinators, communications specialists, and policy bureaucrats who think that mass education is effective. This mass education model – about 5 per cent of the U.S. health budget is spent on health promotion, mostly in relation to healthy living – has been tried at enormous expense for preschoolers, middle schoolers, teens, young adults, new moms, working professionals, and vulnerable groups at risk (for example, single moms on welfare and new immigrants).

The approach is what economists and policy makers refer to as 'soft paternalism' or 'moral suasion.' The special needs of individuals are subverted in favour of mass education. Perhaps this is because the public health sector's historic challenges – clean water, clean air, smoking –

were effectively addressed using broad education campaigns targeting what the public health academy and the policy establishment refer to as 'population-level health' rather than individual health. This bandwagon has been jumped on despite the acknowledged embryonic state of obesity policy research.[81] 'In order to make progress in decreasing the prevalence of obesity, we must shift our view of obesity away from the medical model (which focuses on the individual) to a public health model (which focuses on the population),' states an influential paper in a law journal.[82] Yet the individual model, we argue, is far superior.

Top-down 'megaphone' (also known as 'social marketing') public health policies have clearly worked in reducing levels of smoking, as an example, but they won't work in the case of obesity. The difference is self-evident. No one *has* to smoke, but we all *have* to eat. Since we all need to eat, control over appetite can't be eliminated by diktat. As explained earlier in the book, throughout almost all of human history, mankind's problem has been too little food rather than too much. Accordingly, our bodies are designed to demand food and to pack food away for a rainy day. Our brains have a hard time overruling such signals, even when we know we shouldn't snack, shouldn't nibble, and shouldn't be preparing for famine when the fridge is so close. The body's imperative is to eat, and that makes it hard to stick to a diet. Food brings immediate gratification, while the health costs of overconsumption are delayed. A word to the wise from Rochefoucauld: 'If we resist our passions, it is more because of their weakness than because of our strength.' Free will may not be so free.

A top-down, one-size-fits-all approach is one where governments create 'strategy maps' and 'system goals' prior to implementing a suite of strategies to establish a policy and 'targets' for success. (Example of a public health anti-obesity target: multilingual anti-obesity posters in 90 per cent of state middle schools.) So-called strategy mapping, made famous by management gurus, has become increasingly popular in government circles and in the academy. A top-down 'strategy map' approach to obesity is one that tends to treat any member of a group – a child in a poor school district, a senior citizen, a new mother – more or less in the same way, each as likely as the next to benefit from the same anti-obesity policy. A bottom-up approach, by contrast, is one whose plan or map or goal is set by the individual in a close, sustained collaboration with the individual's primary care provider. It is what has been called 'participatory medicine.'

There is little reason to believe that a 'population health' or 'systems approach' strategy can work to contain the onward march of obesity.

A major 2007 UK government report admitted as much: obesity is a 'complex system,' it concluded, with an individual's energy intake and energy output, and his or her resulting weight, being influenced by a web of factors, many of which remain unknown. Willpower, as we stated earlier, is not sufficient to control our appetites and temptations. Looking at this phenomenon in the context of childhood obesity, a leading clinical epidemiologist summarized the predicament in a *Canadian Medical Association Journal* editorial: 'No simple or short-term changes, such as a physical activity intervention for a limited length of time in the school curriculum, can be expected to influence the prevalence of obesity.'[83]

Adherence to top-down government anti-obesity interventions is fleeting. 'Such an approach,' Louise Baur wrote, 'can be described as "the futility of isolated initiatives."' Unfortunately, Dr Baur's editorial, and the accompanying metareview of failed 'school-based physical activity' interventions (that is, a summary of all academic analyses on the topic of fighting obesity), suggested that the best public policy solution lies in investing *more* tax dollars in longer, more intense, one-size-fits-all initiatives of the very same sort that have so far fizzled. That review's conclusion, with which we disagree, was that these failed initiatives, in order to work, need to be maintained or expanded. That's the same reasoning that rationalizes why diets don't work – because they're not maintained. But maybe there's more to it. Maybe it's not the right public policy diet.

The very complexity of human obesity undermines the one-size-fits-all public health policy approach and almost certainly ensures its failure. We need to be humble about this problem. We actually don't know what will work to constrain obesity to 1980 levels. *And neither does anyone else – not even the First Lady*, who led the 2010 White House Task Force on Childhood Obesity, with input from 12 federal agencies. We believe that there are 6.8 billion potential solutions that every person on the planet will have to explore to see what works for them. We need to fuel bottom-up, small-scale experimental innovations tailored to individual needs and choices, instead of resorting to big-government, top-down approaches. But how do we do this? In chapter 4, we will present a new policy idea – 'Healthy Living Vouchers' – to fight obesity in a way that recognizes and acknowledges individual differences in how we all gain or lose weight. Before we discuss our policy idea, however, let's spend time addressing the one-size-fits-all public health approach.

Personal Struggles, Public Solutions

If you show a picture of one hundred young women to an eighteen-year-old girl suffering from anorexia and ask her to pick her ideal from among the bunch, whom would she pick? She would pick the one who, to non-anorexics, looks emaciated. Now ask a group of non-anorexic men and women to select ideal silhouettes of women's figures. Women's choices are significantly thinner than men's. Many highly educated women throughout Asia go as far as to swallow parasites so that they can weigh less than the magic figure of one hundred pounds, no matter their height – an irrational goal that is fuelling the spike in eating disorders. Why is this? Is it because we are all pawns of psychological illusions, historical and cultural gender biases, and intense social pressures that play on our senses? This certainly applies to us, the authors. We did not come to write on the topic of obesity and choice by accident. We have both struggled with our waist size, and we know, by dint of the evidence on obesity rates, that most of our readers have, too.

Writing this book was a challenge: besides battling weight, we both also fought procrastination when it came to putting pen to paper. How, then, did we ever complete this book, meet the deadline, and keep our friendship intact? We have both written newspaper columns – these are like fast-food snacks. And academic journal articles – gourmet foods · that few people ever read. A policy book with a new idea is meant to be accessible to a wide audience, edible but indelible. Committing to writing such a book is analogous to committing publicly to losing weight – to exposing yourself so that your friends can see your success, or, quite possibly, your failure. The final glorious result beckons, but getting there? How does one start? The process can be immobilizing.

So we entered into a small bet. We split a tiny sum of money evenly and then stipulated the following conditions: whichever of us shed the greater percentage of his body weight prior to book completion would owe the other his portion of the money. Despite this, one of us (the economist) first gained weight. As the deadline for the book's delivery to the publisher loomed, the economist took up jogging. The other (the health policy researcher) lost 30 per cent of his body weight, but was motivated to do so by considerations far removed from the bet itself. He'd fallen in love at age thirty-nine with the sport of boxing and had helped start an inner-city boxing club for professionals – something that was unexpected, impossible to predict. This is a common thread in stories of sustained weight loss. They never fit a pat storyline of 'diet and exercise.'

While this book is not about diets, it is worth noting that in the public mind, a 'good' diet implies that it's good for all. New research shows that genetic swab tests revealing an individual's specific genotype will one day be able to tell whether or not he or she is predisposed to lose weight on a low-carb, high-protein diet (most famously, the 'Atkins diet') or on a diet with some balanced ratio of calories obtained from carbohydrates, proteins, and fats (famously, the 'Zone diet' or 'Ornish diet'). Genetics tells us convincingly that success in weight loss is an individual matter. Endocrinologists and nutrition experts around the world are excited by the accumulating evidence of a genetic predisposition to successful dieting. The evidence helps make a convincing case that diets will only work if we match individuals with highly targeted interventions. From a public policy perspective, we are excited by this research, since it is revolutionizing our understanding of the limited power of public health messaging and providing insight into new policy ideas that incorporate 'matching' and 'targeting.'

Stories of sustained healthy eating and exercise habits appear to be unique to the individual and subject to a good deal of randomness.[84] *Suum cuique* (to each his own), recommended Cicero, who also said – public health promoters, pay heed – that 'advice is judged by results, not by intentions.'

Why Public Health Needs to Change

Public health research has as its ethos the idea of delivering social value or 'system impact,' rather than individual impact. Men and women promoted as leaders in public health and in government are 'system planners,' not personal coaches. Sometimes they are clinicians, and if so, they tend to leave and go back to clinical work. Most are public advocacy coordinators and communications specialists, not individual mentors or field nurses. So, on the topic of healthy eating, many public health research institutes and advocacy groups are committed to shaping public attitudes; individuals are not their chief concern.

In 1920, Charles-Edward Armory Winslow defined public health as 'the science and art of preventing disease, prolonging life and promoting health through the organized efforts and informed choices of society, organizations, public and private, communities and individuals.'[85] If you read the mission statement today of many leading schools of public health, the last bit, the part about 'individuals,' is absent or relegated to second fiddle. And according to one of the websites of the American Association of Public Health, many more system planners are needed. System planners are defined as public health officials whose goals are as follows: improving health, improving accessibility to health services, and promoting efficiency in the provision of services and resources on a comprehensive basis for a whole community. Again, no mention of individuals.

The top-ranked schools of public health make little mention of individuals in their strategic documents. The Johns Hopkins Bloomberg School of Public Health 'is dedicated to the education of a diverse group of research scientists and public health professionals, a process inseparably linked to the discovery and application of new knowledge, and through these activities, to the improvement of health and prevention of disease and disability around the world.' Similarly to Johns Hopkins, the Harvard School of Public Health makes no reference to the distinctiveness of individuals that Winslow saw as essential. Harvard's mission highlights the importance of creating 'a strong and vibrant intellectual community'; training 'leaders in public health science and practice to solve public health problems of the twenty-first century'; and furthering 'new discoveries that lead to improved health for the people of this country and all nations.' Public health today concerns itself with research into system policy, not individual behaviour change.

More problematic, as psychiatrist Sally Satel chronicled in *PC, MD: How Political Correctness Is Corrupting Medicine*, is that public health leaders lobby for '*social* change.'[86] For example, she notes, Ronald Bayer of Columbia University refers to colleagues who believe that 'public health officials can do little or nothing to change the prevailing patterns of morbidity and mortality in the absence of social change.' A former dean of the Harvard School of Public Health, Harvey Feinberg, has said that 'a school of public health is like a school of justice.' Schools of public health, whose leaders' educational training has been in topics such as biostatistics, epidemiology, and water sanitation, now proclaim, according to the AUPHA action plan, that they are in the business of addressing poverty, social injustice, and health disparities that may contribute to the development of terrorism; providing humanitarian assistance to those affected by terrorism; and promoting non-violent means of conflict resolution. These are laudable goals, but they sit outside the ken of public health researchers and public health educational leaders. Furthermore, to the extent that students of public health are learning about these topics in school, they are moving further and further away from enabling individuals to take better care of themselves. This is what we see as the essence of policy failure when it comes to obesity: too much attention has been paid to sweeping social change, and too little attention to what individuals can do to address their own individual obesity challenges. In its early days, public health was about educating people to cough into their sleeves and wash their hands to prevent the spread of infection. It was about immunization and boiling water and using condoms properly. It was, and is, important to teach men how to put on a condom. It's also important to teach people weight management options that suit their individual needs, and ones they can afford.

A lack of attention to individual differences in weight gain and prevention has led to a maze of policy incoherence. In the North American policy community, we are witnessing a mad policy scramble to 'do something,' *anything*, about what is often referred to as the 'silver tsunami' of aging, overweight, obese boomers. Expensive city-, state-, and country-wide policies are steamrolling forward, despite the paucity of evidence that any of these proposed one-size-fits-all anti-obesity policies have even a minuscule chance of success. In 2007, at a meeting of the National Cancer Institute, obesity policy was considered and the following themes emerged: (1) obesity policy research is in its infancy; (2) the outcomes of policy-based efforts to address the obesity epidemic need to be documented and analysed; (3) research focused *beyond individual-level behaviour* change is important, especially economic research; and (4) this policy arena calls for urgent action.[87] Since then, schools around the world have either banned, or are on the verge of banning, sugary drinks; many lawmakers have subsidized 'urban farms'; New York City has passed 'green cart legislation' to increase the number of food carts offering fresh fruits and vegetables to residents of low-income neighbourhoods; and cities like Los Angeles and Berkeley have limited the concentration of fast-food restaurants in low-income areas. So much for individual-level behaviour change. So much for evidence-based policy making.

The U.S. Senate Finance Committee announced in 2009 that it was considering imposing a national tax on sodas and other sweetened beverages.[88] In Maine, the State Legislature approved new wholesale taxes on sodas and the sugary syrup used to make them. In San Francisco, Mayor Gavin Newsom floated the idea of charging big retailers who sell sugary drinks a new fee. Yet countries like Sweden actually saw an *increase* in obesity after banning sugary drink ads in media to which children were exposed.[89]

Under President Barack Obama's new health legislation, there are rules requiring restaurant chains to post calorie counts on their menu boards, copying laws in Massachusetts, California, Philadelphia, and New York City. In Ontario, more than thirty-five municipalities and three school boards have passed resolutions in support of menu labelling. Many cities are banning trans fats, even though these fats constitute a tiny percentage of our caloric intake. Mayor Bloomberg of New York is seeking to have manufacturers reduce their use of salt – and the nutrition panel advising the FDA on the new guidelines similarly recommends reducing salt intake to a maximum of 1,500 milligrams daily. Though some will benefit from reduced salt intake, others won't. Salt is a core part of our diet. Regulating salt intake in manufactured products, with unclear evidence of the system impact, is jumping the gun.

Few bureaucrats stop to think of the personnel costs involved in enforcing these laws. It costs millions of dollars to change labelling, to educate the public about new dietary guidelines, and to regulate manufacturers who create products exceeding state-sanctioned sodium limits. Beware the food police policy bandwagon. Independent evaluations show that dietary guidelines and the posting of calorie counts do not change how much people eat or the types of foods they eat. People who respond positively to lists of calorie counts are already taking excellent care of their health. The majority of Americans are against taxing 'bad' foods; they believe in personal responsibility and not in food police who practise a form of social engineering. 'I don't need the White House or Michelle Obama passing laws telling people applesauce is healthful,' Paul Wroten of Knouse Foods, a Peach Glen, Pennsylvania–based producer of apple sauce, juice, and pie fillings, told reporters following the May 2010 White House task force proposal led by the First Lady.

The First Lady wants to 'talk more' about obesity, yet this can be perceived as little more than feel-good sloganeering. Here is how Dr Regina M. Benjamin, the current U.S. Surgeon General, described the First Lady's campaign to curb obesity, an approach she endorses:

> I want to change the talk from negative conversations about obesity and illness to positive conversations about being healthy and fit, *so basically just shifting the perceived issue and how we look at it*. [Emphasis added.] We've looked at the medical model, and now it's got to become a lifestyle model.

We need to start positive conversations about doing things because people enjoy the activities and doing things because they have fun.

So she told *Healthcare Quarterly* in 2010 (vol. 13, no. 3). ·

Consider a top-down policy currently very much in fashion: banning soft drink sales in elementary schools. Does this really reduce how much soda children drink? We don't think so. Researchers have compared the soft drink consumption of children at schools where it is sold with that of children where it is not sold.[90] About 4 per cent fewer children from the no-soda schools said they avoided it during school hours. But this 4 per cent differential cannot be attributed to the ban. To assess this issue properly, one would have to measure two equal school populations – in location, age, sex, ethnicity, and wealth – and compare one school that did not ban soda, with one that did, over the same time period. One would need to use independent observers to study the children, not just ask the children about their habits. 'This approach is not really solving the problem,' said the author of the definitive study on the topic. So why are the U.S. Senate, countries across Europe, and every state in the United States and province in Canada contemplating a full-scale soda ban? When trans fats were banned in New York, Philadelphia, and other cities, substitutes were brought in that were, in some cases, *higher* in saturated fats. If you eat more of a 'good' food, you still put on the calories. Eliminating or taxing tasty foods may help some people a little, but it's bad policy; it is not Pareto-efficient (that is, making society better off than before).

Dubious Claims of Top-Down Policy Success

On 28 May 2008, the U.S. Centers for Disease Control and Prevention published a bombshell article in the prestigious *Journal of the American Medical Association* suggesting that rates of childhood obesity in the United States had levelled off. A reporter for the *New York Times* wrote: 'It is not clear whether the lull in childhood weight gain is permanent or even if it is the result of public efforts to limit junk food and increase physical activity in schools.'[91]

Could this be the public health establishment's greatest achievement since John Snow identified the Broad Street Pump as the source of the London cholera outbreak in 1854?

After a twenty-five-year hike in child obesity rates, with childhood diabetes rates shooting straight up and other diet-related complications on an apparently inexorable climb, here was a story saying that the obesity epidemic had perhaps reached a plateau; what's more, public health campaigns and system-level planning may have had something to do with it – or so the media storyline went. In North America and around the globe, the story was the most widely read academic news item on obesity reported in the major media in 2008. Dr David Ludwig, director of the childhood obesity program at the prestigious Children's Hospital in Boston, called it a 'glimmer of hope.'

Can the flattening rate of growth in childhood obesity be credited to public health campaigns – essentially, to scattered pilot projects such as anti–junk food posters now peeling off the walls in urban high school hallways; recent bans on soda pop machines in some schools; and mandated twenty-minute physical exercise regimens in inner-city schools? They may have some impact among some kids, but not much, by all accounts. A recent National Bureau of Economic Research study by John Cawley, Chad Meyerhoefer, and David Newhouse has found that while state physical education requirements can make children more active, they have no detectable impact on teenagers' BMIs or their probability of becoming overweight.[92] Yet public health advocates will not give up such 'get moving' approaches: recall the 2010 insight from Jeff Levi, head of the Trust for America's Health, whose organization found weight gain escalating across America yet who attributed one statistically negligible annual drop in the District of Columbia to the expansion of community recreation centres and public transit – expansions that have been taking place in dozens of other states without any slowing in their obesity trend lines.

Just a year before the *JAMA* study came out, in 2007, the influential Institute of Medicine, part of the U.S. National Academy of Sciences, recommended that junk foods such as potato chips, doughnuts, chocolate-covered ice cream, and sugary drinks be banned from all elementary, middle, and high schools.[93] According to the IOM, only through mandated national standards in every single school in America could we make a dent in the problem of childhood obesity. So how was it possible that a year after the IOM announcement, on the heels of the widely cited *JAMA* study, the *New York Times* was speculating on whether public health bureaucrats had won a major battle by halting the rise in childhood obesity? Was the public health establishment guilty of self-interest in claiming credit for 'success'?

In statistical terms, the data from the original *JAMA* study likely resulted from the fact that all major ascents eventually plateau. Also in

2008 and 2009, violent crime rates reached half-century historic lows in cities like Los Angeles and New York. It is now generally accepted that demographic trends – notably an aging population with fewer young people in the younger age category most prone to commit violent crime – explain the phenomenon of declining crime rates. It is rarely the case that abrupt statistical changes in the prevalence of social ills – from obesity to violent urban crime – can be attributed to policy rather than to nature. Americans were all aging at one point and all were growing taller, but then the rate of aging and the rate of growth ebbed. Did this signify success in the control of 'height gain'? Even the rise in obesity has a natural plateau.

That there are ebbs from this peak (as suggested by the *JAMA* data) is statistically meaningless. There's a point at which society – America being a good example – won't get fatter, but that should not be considered 'good news.' Seldom reported in news articles about the *JAMA* study was a quote from the lead author of the report, Dr Cynthia Ogden, who thinks that we may have reached 'some sort of saturation in terms of the proportion of the population who are genetically susceptible to obesity.'[94] This is an example of how data can be interpreted and 'spun' in a variety of ways.

For instance, a National Bureau of Economic Research study by Patricia Anderson and Kristin Butcher concluded that a 10 per cent increase in the availability of junk food was correlated with about a 1 per cent higher BMI for the average student.[95] However, the effect of the junk food appeared strong only for students whose parents were overweight. Researchers from the Karolinska Institute in Sweden conducted a four-year study called STOPP (Stockholm Obesity Prevention Project), in the course of which sweets, buns, and soft drinks were banned from five schools but not from five others. The proportion of overweight six- to ten-year-olds dropped by 3 per cent in the schools with the ban, while it *climbed* by 3 per cent in the schools with no ban.[96] This improvement was encouraging, but child obesity across Sweden was still rising. A review of school-based obesity prevention problems in 2008 stated that out of fourteen such studies, the evidence was weak in ten. The authors concluded:

> Our ability to draw strong conclusions as to the efficacy of school-based obesity prevention programs is limited by the small number of published studies and by methodological concerns. Qualitative analysis suggests programs grounded in social learning may be more appropriate for girls,

while structural and environmental interventions enabling physical activity may be more effective for boys. High-quality evaluation protocols should be considered essential components of future programs.[97]

The only other major 'good news' media-reported study to have appeared in the past few years comes from the NPD Group, a Port Washington, New York–based market research firm. The story, widely circulated in the international media in 2009, contended that the eating habits of American children were changing.[98] 'And for a change, the news is good,' celebrated the *New York Times*. The NPD is one of many major marketing companies skilled at getting reporters to pay attention to their sound-bite stories, and when it comes to teens and obesity, reporters always pay attention. The story in the 'Science Desk' section of the *Times* was titled: 'Kid Goes into McDonald's and Orders … Yogurt?' This is what journalists call a 'man-bites-dog' story; as such, it made news.

The NPD data found that chicken nuggets, burgers, fries, and colas remained popular with the teenage set, but that consumption of these foods was declining, whereas consumption was on the rise for soup, yogurt, fruit, grilled chicken, and chocolate milk. Let's put aside the fact that there are heavily caloric restaurant yogurts, soups, fruits (say, with granola), spicy grilled chicken (usually accompanied by cheesy, crouton-laced Caesar salads), and chocolate milk; are public health campaigns responsible for this 'good news'? NPD analysts insisted that the global economic meltdown in 2008 and 2009 (and the resultant decline in restaurant orders for kids' meals) could not explain the shift, since the costs of healthier foods are comparatively on the rise. Bonnie Riggs of the NPD said that 'kids' tastes and preferences are changing.' Most parents of teenagers would find this astounding.

Left out of the media stories was the fact that young people between eighteen and twenty-four had been eating more at 'fast casual' chains, which are just as caloric. Fast casual chains had simply lowered their prices and spruced up their offerings to draw away calorie-craving customers from Taco Bell, Burger King, McDonald's, and Wendy's. Yet public health opinion leaders jumped on the story as proof of the power of big-government social messaging to promote healthy weights. Leann Birch of the Center for Childhood Obesity told the *Times:* 'The food industry is always saying, "We're giving people what they want; that's why we're giving you chicken nuggets, burgers and fries for your kids." That's not really true. If kids are given different options and if parents make them available and let them choose some of those things, I think quite often we see you do get shifts in eating.'[99] To be sure, kids' tastes are malleable. Parents are an important part of the equation because what they feed their kids early on will program their taste buds for many years to come. And what parents feed their children depends, to a large degree, on how much money they have to spend on healthy food. But none of this means that the public health policy establishment has been somehow responsible for the statistical plateau in childhood obesity reported by the NPD.

'Holistic' Strategies

In thirty-one American states, more than one in four adults are obese, according to a 2009 report from the Trust for America's Health and the Robert Wood Johnson Foundation. No state experienced a decline in obesity from the prior year. Yet strangely, the trust's researchers' policy suggestion to address this crisis was to provide integrated system-wide solutions, not individual ones. 'The obesity epidemic clearly goes beyond being an individual problem,' said Jeff Levi, the trust's executive director.[100] Robert Wood Johnson's vice-president, Dr James Marks, added that the epidemic was a national crisis that 'calls for a national strategy to combat obesity.'

Government officials in a number of countries are pursuing these kinds of 'holistic' strategies. What does this gobbledygook mean? In many cases, an 'integrated strategy' is one that involves enlisting entire communities to fight childhood obesity. The public health 'holistic strategy' had its genesis in France in 1992, with 'Epode' – a French acronym for 'Together Let's Prevent Childhood Obesity.' According to observational research, community-based 'holistic approaches' – which include everything from organized walk-to-school days to government-funded sports activities, chefs in nursery schools, sports educators, and dieticians to counsel children and families in schools – have been effective in two small towns in France. Yet their success is undocumented in the many other towns – from Spain to Belgium to Greece – that have tried them. And these are expensive, taxpayer-funded strategies. The *real* lesson to be gleaned from the two successful northern French towns, Fleurbaiz and Laventie, has escaped many public health officials. It was not the 'holistic strategy' that made the difference, but rather the fact that in these very small towns, families were offered a plethora of new weight loss choices that could work for them, and that after researching them, they chose one. The fact that the *choice was theirs* appears to have been essential.

What to Do about Mississippi (and Places Like It)?

Mississippi, as mentioned earlier in the book, is ground zero on the obesity battlefront. The most recent CDC data (undeniably conservative figures, as they are based on self-reports) suggest that 34.4 per cent of that state's population is obese. The public health plan is to shave that number. Meanwhile, a recent 2009 state 'happiness index' indicates that obese southern states like Mississippi and Louisiana are happiest by all objective measures (New Yorkers are the unhappiest), which suggests perhaps that eating plentifully is a pleasurable activity, or that happy people tend to partake in festive eating more than sad people.

Mississippi House Bill 282, introduced by Republican John Read in that state's House of Representatives in late January 2008, was an act to prohibit designated food establishments from serving food to any person who is obese, as per criteria determined by the Mississippi State Department of Health.[101] In Mississippi, one might think therefore that thin, power-crazed public health bureaucrats run the world. To be fair, Read's position was considered to be on the policy fringe: the state's public health association is committed to what it deems to be more important causes, such as emergency preparedness and epidemiological research. The State Department of Health, like other public health departments across North America, focuses on delivering anti-obesity educational flyers, not on depriving people of food.

A similar proposal to Read's made waves around the same time in Britain, where hoteliers got so worked up by the obese in their midst that they proposed charging fat children extra for Sunday lunch. Youngsters were to be asked to step on the scales to see how much their restaurant meal should cost. A child weighing 70 pounds would pay £5, while a youngster who tipped the scales at 140 pounds would have to shell out £10. Executives at five-star Oulton Hall near Leeds claimed that the idea was 'just a bit of fun.' Child obesity experts condemned it as demeaning, holding, as it did, youngsters up to ridicule. The proposed scheme died. Managers at Oulton Hall, owned by De Vere Hotels, defended it, though spokesman Nigel Massey admitted: 'There will no doubt be people who say it's not politically correct.'[102]

Back in Mississippi, Read's bill introduced a new front in the war on obesity: it exposed XXLs publicly as sinners. Encountering resistance to his idea from an advocacy group for the obese, he back-pedalled, saying that he never intended the bill to become law but had simply wanted to 'raise public awareness' about the severe obesity problem ravaging his state.

What kind of idea was that – denying food to the obese, like a bartender who refuses drinks to a tipsy person? Ridiculously punitive and counterproductive, we would say. For most of us, going out to eat is a pleasure – which might explain why people in heavier, southern states are generally a happy lot. We know we'll put on weight, yet we make a rushed mental calculation – pleasure against pounds – and determine, in the here-and-now moment, that the expected gain in pleasure outweighs the future potential cost of putting on weight. Award-winning behavioural economists have pointed out that human beings consistently pick the bird in the hand: pleasure. Most of us are what economists call 'present biased' in our pleasure preferences, and will be forever so. We get understandably upset at those who stand in the way of our pleasure. And this is why Read retreated.

'It's got people all over stirred up,' Read said. 'Nobody was trying to hurt anybody's feelings here. If anyone's feelings did get hurt, I apologize. Anybody with any sense knows it's not going to happen, not going to pass.'

The bill would have directed the state's Health Department to provide restaurants with written criteria for spotting obese people and would have monitored restaurants to make sure they were abiding by the prohibition. The restaurants would have presumably lost money, but that's legitimate, some might contend. After all, they are complicit in fanning the obesity epidemic; they are the ones hawking twenty-two-ounce rib-eyes, potato skins, and red-glazed cheesecake.

Read had the last word: 'With all the attention paid to tobacco problems, this was to shed some light on another major problem. This has been at least getting the dialogue going.' The dialogue has indeed accelerated, and these are the elements of that dialogue now: Is obesity a sin, a product of sloth and gluttony that needs to be shamed out of existence? Or is it a disability that must be compassionately treated? Alternatively, is it an addiction that requires tough love? Is it all the fault of commercial interests, and should we be gunning for them, making them pay? Is it personal behaviour to be dealt with privately, or should the government step in? If so, when, and with what policy arsenal?[103]

Shaming the Obese?

A high-ranking British public health civil servant recently recommended that the government provide an emergency distress telephone line for overweight people to be emblazoned on all XXL articles of clothing. A new video by the European Union and the Union of European Football Associations depicts the obese as miserable, listless, and helpless. This is mild stuff compared to a public health school policy in Australia, where thousands of children are routinely hauled to the side, weighed, measured, and interviewed about their diet. This is part of that country's much-touted 'national plan' to tackle obesity. Meanwhile, students at Lincoln University in Pennsylvania with a BMI of 30 or above must take a fitness course three hours per week. Those assigned to the class cannot graduate unless they complete it.

In 2007 the City of Boston spent $250,000 on a childhood obesity ad campaign. One ad shows an overweight child on a scale with the caption 'Fat Chance.' Another billboard shows the flabby back of an overweight child and asks: 'If that's your kid, what are you waiting for?' The New York City Health Department recently ran an ad that shows a cola being poured over a glass of human fat, with this caption: 'Are you pouring on the pounds?'

A shaming mentality is circulating throughout the public health movement and across popular culture around the world. Overweight people are harming the planet as well as their own bodies, according to Sir Jonathan Porritt, chairman of the UK's Sustainable Development Commission.[104] He is on a bizarre public campaign, insisting that 'fat is a climate change issue.' Overweight people eat more protein-rich food, such as beef or lamb, than the rest of us, he said in 2009; this in turn is responsible for producing greenhouse gases because of the methane emitted by livestock. So, like smokers, the obese are harming not only themselves directly, but all of us indirectly.

In the fall of 2007, the Ad Council and the U.S. Department of Health and Human Services released two hard-hitting ads to raise awareness of obesity: the first ad consisted of two children poking at a belly discarded by someone walking on the beach; the second was of a man pulling his dog away from another discarded body part – this time a pair of buttocks shed by a parent playing with children in a playground.

In a public health campaign to 'help Aussies lose weight,' AirAsia X is considering charging its passengers according to their weight. Dr John Tindrell, a leading Australian nutritionist, has been lobbying for an airline tax for some time.[105] 'I fly Sydney to Perth – five hours – and being totally disadvantaged by some huge person next to me literally flopping over into my seat. Why should I pay the same as them?' he told the BBC in 2007. Most major airlines are monitoring trends in the size and shape of their customers. Air France has been an industry leader: in 2009 it began charging obese passengers a double fare. This, even though the airline was ordered two years earlier to pay £5,000 in damages to an obese passenger who had his stomach measured at an airport check-in desk before being told to buy two seats.

Airlines have alleged special needs because of the implications of weight for safe takeoff. In early 2009, UAL Corp.'s United Airlines joined Southwest Airlines Co. and several other carriers in implementing a formal policy to demand that obese customers buy two seats. Speaking to the *Wall Street Journal*, Willis Reed, a credit union vice-president, said: 'Airlines mandate that carry-ons have to fit certain sizes, so why not passengers? I was just sitting there thinking, the company paid for me to sit here, but what do I get? Do I surcharge them for encroaching on my seat?' Trouble is, the two-seat solution is difficult to enforce owing to safety issues with current seatbelt design. Tall passengers butt their knees up against the seat in front of them; teenagers bang away on their loud Game Boys and other gadgets; babies scream; drunken passengers use foul language. Should the obese be singled out for special attention? Isn't this inherently discriminatory?

Right before Christmas of 2009, New York City officials released a campaign of shock videos, which were virally marketed over YouTube. One of these videos showed a man gorging on liquefied fat, in a full-on attack aimed at discouraging the consumption of sugary drinks. The fat-guzzling video has been all the rage in the public health policy establishment.[106] 'Sugary drinks shouldn't be a part of our everyday diets,' said New York health commissioner Thomas Farley.[107] Michael Jacobson, executive director for the Center for Science in the Public Interest, a U.S. public health advocacy group, applauded the move. Touting the brave leadership of New York's health department, he recommended that other countries, notably Canada, 'look very closely at what New York City is doing' to expose fatties.

In 2008, Japanese public health officials unveiled an anti-obesity law that mandates employers to measure the waistlines of employees between forty and seventy-four years of age – approximately 44 per cent of the working population.[108] Men cannot exceed a waistline of 33.5 inches, and women cannot exceed 35.4 inches. Failure to abide by the limits leads to fines and dieting assistance. A Japanese commentator explained: 'Nobody will want to be singled out as [obese]. It'll have the same effect as non-smoking campaigns where smokers are now looked at disapprovingly.'

When obesity is framed as a lack of personal responsibility or will-power, this translates into stigma against the obese. Doctors internalize this shaming mentality as well. They see their obese patients as unmotivated or lazy. The heavier patients are, the less respectfully they're treated. One study described obese patients as 'awkward, unattractive, ugly, and unlikely to comply with treatment.'[109] This is unfortunate, because these patients may end up avoiding the health care system altogether. Physician biases simply mirror the prejudices that obese persons are subjected to in other settings – in the workplace, for example, they tend to be paid less and promoted more slowly. A recent study by Dalton Conley and Rebecca Glauber of New York University found that a 1 per cent increase in a woman's BMI results in a 0.6 per cent decrease in her family income – that's a pretty large effect – and a 0.4 per cent decrease in her occupational prestige, both measured thirteen to fifteen years later.[110] The obese report experiencing weight-related stigma in a wide range of environments, especially at work. There is well-documented discrimination in media portrayals, in education, and in housing opportunities.[111]

A government's posture on obesity influences how citizens in general and health care workers in particular perceive overweight people. When the overweight are held exclusively accountable for keeping trim but aren't given any viable options or any financial means to do it, it legitimizes public ridicule, which is growing in intensity across the West. In the United States, the courts and federal laws do not protect obese people from discrimination. Only one state, Michigan, bans discrimination on the basis of weight. (Dr Delos M. Cosgrove, a cardiac surgeon and CEO of the Cleveland Clinic, told the *New York Times* in 2009 that if he could get away with it legally, he would refuse to hire anyone who is obese.[112] In fact, he *can* get away with it, and many CEOs and managers do.) The reported prevalence of weight discrimination is today suddenly on par with rates of racial discrimination. And for adults, being on the receiving end of anti-obesity barbs has been associated, in study after study, with profound depression, anxiety, low self-esteem, suicidal behaviour, binge eating, unhealthy eating – and, significantly, the *avoidance* of physical activity and health care services.[113] Psychologists June Tangney and Ronda Dearing, in their book

Guilt and Shame, document the fact that feelings of shame (in contrast to guilt) promote self-destructive behaviours, attempts to escape very painful feelings of shame. They could not detect any apparent benefit from shaming. Shaming does not deter young people from crime or from unsafe sexual practices or unsafe driving habits.

A study by John Cawley of Cornell University reports that heavy white women – but not black women or men – are paid less than their counterparts. He finds that among white women, an increase of two standard deviations in weight – that's about sixty-five pounds – is associated with wages dropping by 9 per cent. Assuming that this relationship reflects cause and effect, it implies that losing sixty-five pounds has about the same labour market impact as an extra eighteen months of education.

The West, as represented by its leaders, is today personified as limber and svelte. In the past, global leaders from Henry VIII to Winston Churchill were remarkably rotund. Today we disproportionately elect wealthy, slim leaders. Our leaders are athletes, while our fellow citizens keep getting fatter. French President Nicolas Sarkozy keeps to a gruelling jogging regimen. President Obama leads the G-20 pack of leader-athletes. He endures intense cardio sessions. President George W. Bush before him was a hard-driving cyclist. The UK's David Cameron, the newly elected prime minister, also bikes, and the once portly Gordon Brown, now out of 10 Downing Street, very publicly took up pilates. So there is a noticeable divide between the leader (slim) and the populace (fat).

Consider the case of Singapore, which claims to have enjoyed great success in its battle against childhood obesity.[114] Prime Minister Lee Hsien Loong, an alumnus of the country's armed forces and of the U.S. Army Command and General Staff College at Fort Leavenworth, is a model of fitness. His government is on a public health campaign to mould its citizens in similar fashion. Over the past fifteen years, the proportion of obese children in that country has dropped from 14 per cent to 9 per cent. Their approach in 'Trim and Fit' clubs has been to single out overweight children for insult and embarrassment, to mandate their participation in daily strenuous exercise, and to give them fewer 'calorie coupons' to spend at lunch than are provided to their slimmer friends. Targeted children are openly mocked and insulted into changing their behaviour.

Some former Trim and Fit club members say the act of segregation and labelling motivated them to change. Is it worth it? Singapore psychologist David Kan, who has tracked the medical consequences for those affected, says that past members of these clubs are deeply scarred: such shaming and social ostracism have caused palpable harm.[115] And the stigma and bullying are only part of the problem. Worst of all are the messages that get internalized – messages that lead to self-loathing until the participants believe they are not good enough to be part of the club.

All the while, the likely reason for the statistical decline in childhood obesity in Singapore has been not the shaming but a rapid drop in the country's fertility rate and an influx of wealthy, healthy foreigners. In 2006, Singapore's total fertility rate was only 1.26 children per woman, among the lowest in the world and well below the 2.1 population replacement level. In 2006, 38,317 Singaporean babies were born, compared to around 37,600 in 2005. The government had been encouraging very wealthy foreigners to immigrate to Singapore. These large numbers of immigrants to Singapore tend to be at the very top end of the wealth scale, the slim affluent.

Weight is climbing in almost every social and economic class around the world. The sole exception seems to be one very narrow sliver – the top 1 per cent of income earners. Why are the super-rich (that is, those for whom a hundred-foot yacht is not outside the bounds of affordability) thin if much of the variability in weight gain is attributable to genes over which social status has no control? Perhaps in extremely wealthy circles, embarrassment does have impact. The very wealthy – those who summer in Maui, send their children to elite private boarding schools, ski in the Swiss Alps, and take helicopter 'extreme vacations' in the Canadian Rockies – invest more in their appearance than the rest of us do, and they have greater access to reminders of the need to be thin, such as premium weight loss centres and fitness studios, as well as expensive boutiques catering to a young and slim body shape. Most important, the super-rich can afford the leisure time to exercise (one to two hours daily) that most of us cannot. Among the super-wealthy, the overweight really do stand out. Yet to the extent that shame contributes to weight loss, this happens because the super-rich feel pressure from their *peers*, not from the state.

However, many of the policy solutions for combating public health problems – from smoking to AIDS to obesity – hinge on fundamental assumptions about how the public at large will respond to *state-driven* shaming rituals. So here is the question we pose for policy makers: Will taxpayer-funded shaming ever work with the general public in the case of obesity? We suggest that the idea that most people can ever be shamed by the state into eating less and exercising more is not borne out by the evidence. State shaming policies just don't work for obesity. And while many public health policy makers may think that their expensive social marketing campaigns and hot-lunch programs combined with 'healthy choice' messages are benign, they are, in many cases, wasteful and even hurtful system-wide initiatives that keep our eyes off workable, individualized solutions that treat people with dignity and humanity and respect. Treating people with dignity is the first step toward sensible obesity policy; shaming them, and homogenizing them, and treating them as empty-headed targets, undermines all good intentions.

Even when they don't set out to shame, government bully pulpit messages about obesity seem to be about highlighting moral failings. Such stigmatization can misfire and be counterproductive, especially for children: such methods have resulted in unprecedented levels of body hatred in preteen and teenage girls, unhealthy and inappropriate weight loss attempts, fear of food, eating disorders, and nutritional deficits. One can argue that the state telling us to eat our vegetables is not explicitly targeted at the obese and is, therefore, not shaming. Like all discrimination, however, it's the perception that counts. Many obesity policy professionals agree. In a recent article, Rebecca Puhl and Chelsea Heuer concluded: 'On the basis of current findings, the authors propose that weight stigma is not a beneficial public health tool for reducing obesity. It [stigma] generates health disparities, and interferes with effective obesity intervention efforts. These findings highlight weight stigma as both a social justice issue and a priority for public health.'[116]

Perhaps one of the reasons why shame techniques have become so popular is that many facets of commercial activity profit by them. Japan, associated in the public mind with the concept of saving face, now flaunts nudity, flatulence, and partner swapping in TV programming meant to emulate American-style shame-based reality shows. *Love Love Chen* has been a runaway success for the major network TV Nagoya since its debut in May 2005. In one segment, a forty-seven-year-old woman dumps her forty-two-year-old husband for a nineteen-year-old, parading her boy toy around Kyoto in a kimono. Elsewhere, millions of Japanese TV viewers cannot seem to get enough of seeing grown men stripping naked; one national celebrity and reality television contestant, Nasubi, won acclaim for his signature celebratory dance in the buff, televised throughout Japan every Sunday evening.

This Japanese TV genre of humiliation is increasingly popular in America. In an episode of the *Tyra Banks Show,* supermodel Banks donned a fat suit, made herself look as if she weighed 350 pounds, and hopped around on camera eliciting snickers, hoots, and evil sneers from would-be blind dates. In the hit American show *The Biggest Loser,* XXLs are pitted against one another to see who can lose weight the fastest and win the $250,000 prize. The show, despite its protestations to the contrary, appears to us to celebrate rapid and potentially unsafe weight loss. Contenders expose themselves during weigh-ins wearing spandex shorts and bras. They sweat and shed tears. Some viewers empathize, but many more laugh, mocking contestants later online. These shaming tactics may work for some, but it's not a choice we can see many people making.

The Curious Case of Alcohol: Doesn't Shame Sometimes Work?

Shame is an ages-old tool in the armamentarium of public health policy. People in public health, whose job, they feel, is to influence behaviour change at a system level, think of shame – correctly – as a public policy weapon that worked for alcohol abstinence. To understand the success enjoyed by groups like Alcoholics Anonymous (AA), however, one must understand the historical context in which AA was founded. Alcoholics Anonymous was founded more than seventy years ago in the United States, at a time when sobriety was highly esteemed and intemperance was abhorred. Shame was seen as an expedient way to deflate the self-image of boisterous alcoholics and cow them into subservience. The founders observed that exploiting shame stripped away the alcoholic's bombastic persona, allowing for genuine self-reflection and gradual recovery. As a result, AA was able to forge intimate relationships with its pious clients: AA provided group support, solidarity, and community acceptance in exchange for a public disrobing that led to sobriety.

The shame component of AA resonated at first because of its resemblance to popular Victorian mores. Since then, the fact that alcoholism poses grave consequences to the general public when the alcoholic sits behind the wheel of a car or operates heavy machinery has justified the continued use of shaming by public health policy makers. We are all familiar with heavy-hitting anti-drinking campaigns. The most effective are those that describe how utterly shunned the viewer would be if he killed someone else in a drunken crash. The justification of stigma, therefore, is the direct safety risk that alcoholics pose for others. Alcoholics, no matter how addicted, can refrain from driving when they have been drinking. Compare this to obese people, who pose no real health risks for other members of society. They pose *indirect* risk by cutting into scarce health care dollars, but as we shall see later on, it has been argued the obese pay their 'fair share' of medical premiums. And because they work for lower wages, they actually save money for some employers.

Obesity and the Sting of Shame

In Western societies today, extra weight is, by itself, a physical mark of shame; unlike smoking, you cannot mask it with cologne. We all worry about how we measure up to others; shame can be easily induced in most people. When our thoughts are ignored or overridden, when our ideas are dismissed and we're made to feel invisible, we are likely to feel shame, and others, knowing this, can easily take advantage of us. A person who is ashamed of his girth tends to avoid eye contact, turns his head away, and look down. He subtly exits the room when conversation turns to exercise or diet regimens. He looks as if he is trying to hide something, and indeed he is. He is hiding himself. He wants to disappear from the situation that is inducing the shame, and this shows itself in a helpless posture of appeasement or submission. He wants to shrink, literally.

Shame is an emotion elicited by the perception of personal shortcomings involving a sense of public exposure of one's flaws in front of a real or imagined audience. Some people become self-righteous when they feel publicly shamed, and some retaliate by trying, in some way, to belittle those who induce the shame. Shame, let's not kid ourselves, is also a weapon of social control. Public health authorities, with their immense legislative power, such as the power to quarantine during disease outbreaks, are often oblivious to the shame-inducing impact of their education efforts. In the old days, people were placed in village stocks as a means of public shaming. Shaming penalties were alternatives to imprisonment. Today we still try to enforce compliance with public health measures through the inculcation of ever sterner 'healthy living' messages and the threat of public disgrace.

Is More Information the Answer? (or, Why Obesity Is Different from Smoking)

Data that we present in chapter 4 indicate that a large portion of people in North America and in the UK believe that the state's proper role in obesity policy should be that of mere information provider. For many, the public health minister, or surgeon general, or 'health czar,' is a kind of persuader- or moralizer-in-chief. Theoretically, just providing fact-based information could get government out of the shame business – even if providing mere information, like healthy eating messages, fails to do anything meaningful about reducing obesity. But consider: How much *more* information does the public truly need about the dangers of obesity and its attendant risks?

We believe that the public understands full well what puts on weight; and we know what keeps calorie accumulation at bay: more output, less intake. For at least half a century, international health agencies and governments and parents around the world have been reporting on the dangers of obesity. There are many who do not admit publicly to being fat, but every sentient being knows that being fat makes for ill health, not to mention a deeply unpleasant social life.

To be sure, there are important informational items that some people do not know: for example, that bagels and cream cheese are far more loaded with bad stuff than good, or that sugary orange juice can crimp your diet. But these are detail issues. The real problem for the public is less about a gap in access to accurate information than about acting intelligently on what they already know. This makes obesity different from heavy alcohol consumption, and especially from smoking, which required information-packed public health campaigns to brief us on its fatal impact. It wasn't until 1964 that the Surgeon General's Advisory Committee Report on Smoking and Health concluded that tobacco was linked to cancer. That report had a game-changing effect. Science moved the needle on public attitudes; legislation to limit the sale of cigarettes and their use in public places followed.

Today, people widely accept the connection between tobacco and cancer and a wide range of other illnesses. In the 1950s, even highly educated people simply didn't know these basic facts – in 1958, only 44 per cent of Americans saw the link. By the late 1960s, 71 per cent of Americans believed that smoking caused cancer. Americans (and the world) needed to learn about the negative effects of smoking. Keep in mind that cigarette companies sported doctors in white coats on their TV ads until the late 1960s. At the time of writing, smoking is at its lowest rate in North America in more than three decades, yet recent evidence shows convincingly that the lifespan benefits of this down-ward trend in smoking are being eviscerated by the steadily worsen-ing trends in obesity. Obesity is catching up to smoking – some say it has already exceeded it – as the leading, preventable cause of death. A recent study, reported in the *New England Journal of Medicine*, forecast life expectancy and quality-adjusted life expectancy for a representative eighteen-year-old, assuming a continuation of past trends in smoking and in BMI.[117] The negative effects of increasing BMI drowned out the positive effects of declines in smoking. The authors concluded that, if obesity trends continued unchecked, their negative effects on the health of Americans would increasingly outweigh the positive effects of lower smoking rates.

For half a century at least, we have known that soda and chips are bad for us. 'Eat five servings of fruits and vegetables a day.' 'Exercise moderately, at least thirty minutes a day, several times a week.' There's a national U.S. Campaign to End Obesity, which is 'dedicated to reversing America's costliest medical condition' and which lobbies vociferously for 'federal policies that promote healthy weight.' Only a Rip Van Winkle could escape the trumpet call of the state's healthy lifestyle exhortations. For generations, schoolchildren in the fattest jurisdictions in the world – from the American South to the UK to rural India – have learned from their families and communities, from their governments, and from their schools, about good nutrition and choosing snacks carefully. In places like hefty West Virginia, such lessons are part of the core school curriculum. West Virginia and Arkansas, among the heaviest jurisdictions anywhere, ban soft drinks. Yet over the past twenty years the share of Americans between forty and seventy-four who eat five fruits and vegetables a day has *dropped* to 26 per cent from 42 per cent. It is increasingly hard – and in the case of public health advocates, even disingenuous – to make the policy case that throwing more fruits-and-vegetables-and-exercise information at the public – a mainstay of the public health communication policy arsenal – will achieve a lasting positive benefit for society.

Consider just one recent 2009 study in the journal *Obesity*, by Dolores Albarracin, Wei Wang, and Joshua Leeper of the Department of Psychology at the University of Illinois at Urbana-Champaign.[118] They found that promotional state-run messages to exercise actually led to *greater* food intake. Words like 'active' and 'get moving' may subliminally make people think they're exercising when in fact they're not. 'These inadvertent effects may explain the limited efficacy of exercise-promotion programs for weight loss,' the researchers noted. And for some people, purchasing foods with calorie counts stencilled on the package is, as odd as it may seem, close enough to dieting to make them feel that they've paid their dieting dues.

Recent research into consumer psychology shows that shaming, if not handled carefully, can backfire. One recent study suggests that ads focusing on the shamefulness of overdrinking don't change bad drinking habits; instead, they motivate people to drink *more*. 'That's what blows my mind,' said author Nidhi Agrawal of Northwestern's Kellogg School of Management. 'The ads aren't just ineffective … They hurt the very cause you're trying to help.' His study, with Adam Duhachek of Indiana University, looked at an Ontario campaign titled 'Best Night of My Life' that was launched during prom season of 2003. The print ad showed a young woman from behind who has wrapped herself around a toilet bowl to vomit. 'Don't let drinking flush your prom night down the drain,' it warned. In assessing the ad, students said it made them *more* likely to binge drink in the future. They thought the ad would make people want to drink more!

Here's the reality: Most of the top-down messaging campaigns we hear about in the media or in public health conference sessions have not met basic evidence-based standards. Many of the other popular one-size-fits-all public health fads suffer from major logic flaws. Nutritious school lunch programs do not block the entrance to the Wendy's down the street. With most American teenagers taking part-time jobs and easily able to afford fast foods (which are increasingly cheap), school lunch programs should be named 'healthy choice chic.' So maybe it's the corner store that's making children fat, the same corner store that is the epicentre of Western capitalism and that will never disappear. Do we want to kill the corner store and megacorporations (which together employ hundreds of millions of people) by imposing oppressive taxes? No, we don't.

Children who are forced to purchase only healthy meals in the school cafeteria will continue to buy inexpensive candy bars, sugary drinks, and high-sodium snacks elsewhere. School principals told the 2010 White House Task Force on Obesity that serving healthy food that doesn't taste good is a waste of time and money because kids throw it away. Just as relevant is the cost of these healthy lunch programs. Under the U.S. school lunch program, the Department of Agriculture gives public schools cash for every meal they serve – US$2.57 for a free lunch, $2.17 for a reduced-price lunch, and 24 cents for a paid lunch. In 2007 the program cost around $9 billion, a figure widely acknowledged as inadequate to even cover food costs. Very little of the money goes toward food. Schools have to use it to pay for everything from custodial services to heating in the cafeteria. Imagine if this same $9 billion were to go directly to families of U.S. school-aged children. We think they would spend it more effectively than schools do on their children's specific nutritional needs – a topic to which we will return in chapter 4.

Despite lack of evidence of benefit, school lunch advocates are getting bolder. Timothy Cipriano, Executive Director of Food Services for the New Haven public schools, drives a daily truck convoy of entrées to the district's fifty-two schools from a central kitchen.[119] With childhood obesity the chief concern of the district's Wellness Committee, he has replaced chicken patties with 'real chicken' from whole-roasted birds. A typical menu includes chicken stir fry with zucchini and snow peas. Let us hope New Haven succeeds, but the weight of evidence suggests it will not. Fast-food restaurants are inevitably clustered within walking space of high schools. We know that adolescents who go to school within half a mile of a fast-food restaurant are more likely to be overweight or obese than kids whose schools are located farther away. It is not the state's role, nor is it logistically feasible, to uproot fast-food restaurants that happen to be physically close to schools. Nor can schools prevent an entrepreneurial high schooler from purchasing junk food in bulk and reselling it (at a premium) to freshmen – an inevitable phenomenon.

Pity the schools. They are the favourite laboratories for most of today's fashionable public health policy try-outs. But consider an experiment that economist Leonard Epstein and his colleagues ran among a group of middle schoolers.[120] They gave the kids some money and laid out a tray of their favourite junk foods and their favourite healthy snacks. The kids could buy whichever foods they wished. Across groups of students, however, the testers varied the amounts of money that kids were allowed to spend, and also varied the relative prices of the junk foods and healthy snacks. Sometimes the kids had very little money and faced a choice between expensive carrots and cheap chocolate chip cookies. In these circumstances, the kids naturally chose the cookies. When the testers made the junk food items more expensive, the kids still stuck with the junk foods, settling for a smaller number of cookies rather than more of the less expensive apple slices or carrot sticks. The 'elasticity of demand' for foods like carrots is pretty flat when carrots have to compete with tastier fare that gratifies a carbohydrate urge. Epstein's experiment shows that tightening the noose around children's choices – using financial incentives – is a tough slog. Add to this the availability of cheap food to children and it's tempting to declare the war on obesity unwinnable.

The persuasion messages aren't working, so, ironically, some public policy wonks want to make them *more* aggressive. In a *Harvard Business*

Review paper, economist Peter Ubel writes:

> Think about how effective the poison label has been in keeping people from ingesting poisonous materials. The word poison, in large type, would never have had as much impact as that skull and crossbones picture. If we want to discourage Burger King customers from ordering Whoppers, and encourage them to eat the healthier items on the menu, we need to appeal not only to their intellect, but also to their emotions.[121]

The trouble with Ubel's argument is that all evidence we have thus far seen in the obesity field – as opposed to the field of poison control (where ingestion of the poison can kill, and the manufacturer can be held criminally liable for negligent harm or death) – shows that 'danger' labels on fast food don't work (and may actually encourage more unhealthy eating).

To pander to emotion with obesity mass-marketing messages is to fall into the trap that pretends that obesity is the same problem for one person as it is for another. For instance, here is a nuance that is hard for policy makers to grasp, much less message: while obesity kills, being just slightly overweight is often *good* for your health. We know that obesity increases the risk of death from cardiovascular disease, diabetes, and cancers of the colon, breast, esophagus, uterus, and ovary. But being thin is not always a good personal solution because it has been linked to an increased risk of death from non-cancer and non-cardiovascular causes (such as infections or trauma).

The fact is that for some people, being slightly overweight (but not obese) is associated with a *decrease* in the risk of death. The 'fat acceptance' activists therefore have science on their side to a certain extent: we cannot assume that someone is unhealthy just because he's fat, any more than we can assume that someone is healthy just because he's slim. In many cases, epidemiological studies linking weight to disease fail to adjust for non–weight-related risk factors, many of which we're just in the very early stages of discovering. So you can't label food with an obnoxious 'poison' label. One man's poison is another man's potato chip.

Carrying some extra weight in older age allows for nutritional reserves. This comes in handy when fighting infection or recuperating from trauma. One hypothesis – by Jesse Roth, an investigator at the Feinstein Institute for Medical Research in Manhasset, New York – even postulates that fat not only stores energy but also buttresses the body's immune system.[122] Larger people may have enjoyed a survival advantage in the 1800s, when tuberculosis was rampant. Even extreme-ly overweight NFL linemen (typically over three hundred pounds), as reported in the *Journal of the American Medical Association* in 2009, can be at about the same risk of a heart attack as average, healthy young men (presumably because their hearts get a good, regular workout on the football field).[123] Try wrapping these nuances into a simple public health sound bite.

The Psychology of Shaming

Sigmund Freud might have attributed the policy failure around obes-ity to the pleasure principle, which in his view would have precluded any possibility that rational recommendations could ever succeed in changing lifestyles and eating behaviour. Appetites, he would have told us today, come into being in very early preconscious life, so we are unaware of the imperatives that stir our greed. And how can people fight powerful forces of which they are unaware? Not with their will-power, and not with their intellect, which instead of helping, fabricates illusions, elaborates fantasies of wishful thinking, and denies that we consume more than we expend. Who better than Freud to understand that moralizing doesn't stand a chance when we are battling instincts and the pleasure principle? Freud, like us today, would have found it objectionable that current public health policies don't address the importance of pleasure, or happiness. Indeed, they ignore happiness and emphasize its very opposite, shame.

Inspired by Freud, we set about to test the social contagion theory of obesity referred to earlier in the book. We were curious to see how effective online communities of friends were in encouraging peers to lose weight or eat healthy. By the logic of the 2007 *New England Journal of Medicine* study's authors, intimate online peers – mirroring real-life friendships – could positively influence group attitudes toward weight loss.[124] Our analysis revealed that, far from being sites of encourage-ment and inspiration, some of these online communities (certainly not all) have emerged as spew-flecked forums for adult men and women to grouse about their spouses' love handles or to bemoan a girlfriend's or husband's beefiness: a ritual abuse and shaming gallery.

Nowhere is this more prevalent than on YouTube, a massive reposi-tory of videos constituting an interactive community, which is also the third most popular website in the world, reaching almost 20 per cent of all Web users daily.

Here is what our analysis revealed: Of the most downloaded videos about fat people (as of 17 March 2009), more than 90 per cent are hateful attacks on overweight kids and adults – the irony being that, by probabilities, a large majority of those watching the videos must themselves be overweight or obese. In only one of the top ten downloaded videos is obesity looked at seriously; it interviews XXL-sized people in an earnest attempt to document their poignant attempts to lose weight. Notably, this video is deliberately positioned as a *reaction* to the cruelty videos that dominate this website, which is visited by millions of people every day.

The Most Popular YouTube Obesity Videos: A Hall of Shame

YouTube Video Name by Popularity Rank (17 March 2009):

1. Fat People Aren't Funny (an earnest attempt to respond to the animus toward fat people)
2. Fat People Hurt in Funny Accidents Part II ('painful video collection')
3. Fat People USA ('gross florida stuffedpig [sic]')
4. McDonalds™ Makes Fat People ('fat kid dances to Mcdonald's [sic] rap')
5. Fat People Are Beautiful ('pics of different fat people, its funni to watch [sic]')
6. Fat People Are Greedy
7. Fat People Accidents Stunts and Bloopers Compilation
8. Fat People Collection ('fat obese people lol [laugh out loud]')
9. Funny Fat People Video ('fat fatty chubby wow')
10. George Carlin Fat People ('talking about crazy fat people')

The YouTube culture of barbs against fat kids is now played out every day in pretty much every schoolyard around the industrialized world. Comedian Ricky Gervais, not svelte at the time of writing, has jokingly criticized fat people who have surgery to lose weight by saying they should 'stop eating, get off your arse and go for a run.'[125] The star of *The Office* and *Extras* said that people who have liposuction and gastric band operations are 'lazy f---ing fat pigs.' If you are reading this and your child has ever been a fat kid or you are a new mom who can't shed her pregnancy weight, you know this reality too well. When shaming fat people comes by way of TV comedy, is it harmless? Sadly, no.

Researchers in British Columbia distributed a questionnaire to more than 250 people and found that, for many, the very sight of an obese person today triggers disgust; also, those most likely to be disgusted were those who had struggled most with weight gain themselves.[126] Many said they would avoid hiring someone fat. *People* magazine, which once featured the actress Melissa Joan Hart in a bikini and weighing just 113 pounds, now says that her heavier, post-pregnancy self is 'horrifying.' 'The culture rewards that self-disgust,' says Kate Harding, one of the authors of *Lessons from the Fat-o-Sphere: Quit Dieting and Declare a Truce with Your Body.*[127]

It is possible that this revulsion is a built-in response – seeing something out of the norm and therefore not healthy, perhaps contagious ... so better to stay away. Maybe those who stay away have a strong survival instinct. The same people who shudder when they see someone obese also turn away in disgust at someone with a visible rash or mole. Children as young as seven have shown this innate aversion to those who look abnormal, including the abnormally fat. Even parents seem to turn against their obese children, treating them differently from their normal-weight children. They get mad at them for not losing weight when they 'should.'

Discrimination against overweight people is on a dramatic rise, according to a 2008 study by Yale's Rudd Center for Food Policy and Obesity.[128] The information showing that weight discrimination has increased from 7 per cent to 12 per cent came from two waves of the National Survey of Midlife Development in the United States (MIDUS), conducted in 1995–6 and 2004–6. This survey polled nearly 3,500 adults between thirty-five and seventy-four years old. Instances of discrimination that were listed included being denied a scholarship, job, or promotion; losing a job; being denied a bank loan; receiving inferior medical care; being hassled by police; receiving poorer service in a restaurant or store; name calling; threats; and harassment.

Scientific understanding of the rapid growth in stigma attached to obesity is only beginning. Independent observational studies show that obese children are not doing well in school because of the daily harassment from peers. These children report being afraid to walk down the hallways because of negative remarks they receive from schoolmates. Many are ridiculed in physical education classes, teased in the school cafeteria, and humiliated on the bus. A 2008 study asked observers to rank individuals in terms of likeability. Simulation software was used to develop twelve modern figures, using three-dimensional high-resolution images. They depicted one overweight, one non-overweight, and four disabled children of each sex. Two hundred sixty-one children of multiple ethnic backgrounds were recruited from public and private schools to rank these figures in order of likeability. Overweight figures were ranked as significantly less likeable and as less intelligent than the others.[129]

We believe that shaming, name calling, threats, and harassment, common as they now are, indulge a climate of opinion that makes shaming rituals acceptable, logical, and increasingly desirable as public policy tools of choice. When shaming rituals find their way into official public health policy, they may well make things worse. As we noted, even statements sternly advising the public to eat a low-fat diet can have the unintended consequence of fanning the current obesity epidemic.

The costs are high when a society implements shaming policies to combat obesity; the benefits, such as they are, are marginal, effective only for a narrow slice of wealthy, very well educated, highly motivated people. We argue that while there may be a place for shaming in certain policy issues, such as drunk driving or smoking during pregnancy, obesity is not one of them. As we have noted, the power of shaming in influencing eating and weight control is very limited on account of the reality – seldom acknowledged in public policy debates – that the struggle against overeating is intensely individual and private and resistant to one-size-fits-all approaches. Let us now test these observations by taking a short tour of the current politics of obesity.

From Thought to Action

Canada is aiming, at a cost of tens of millions of dollars, to set nationwide standards, policies, and ongoing marketing for nutritious meals and snacks for Canadian children. To set such standards is not to shame, but the very notion of standards reflects the one-size-fits-all public health mantra. Other industrialized countries either already have such standards in place or are embarking upon them. Do they do any good?

Even individuals who know they are at immediate risk for diabetes, fatal heart attacks, or stroke, and adults with high cholesterol levels, do not readily implement changes to their diet, changes that they should rationally know will prolong their lives. A recent survey of four hundred U.S. adults with high cholesterol found that nearly everyone (95 per cent) agreed that a change in diet and regular exercise would be the right way to lower cholesterol.[130] Yet only half were doing anything about it (that is, half said they were). This may be explained by the larger reality described in much of the marketing literature, perhaps best summed up by Martin Lindstrom in his 2008 book *Buyology: Truth and Lies about Why We Buy*.[131] Lindstrom notes that, fundamentally, people are not rational in their purchasing decisions; they make product selection decisions based almost 85 per cent of the time on emotions, habit, superstition, and impulse.[132] Food purchases, we feel, fall entirely into this 85 per cent bracket since our attachment to food is deeply emotional, especially for the depressed. To break through this emotional attachment requires very powerful incentives that uniquely draw on the history and circumstances of the individual, not those of society in general.

Why are people so fundamentally reticent to move from thinking about losing weight to acting on the thought?[133] As game theorists such as Merrill Flood have observed, people are, predictably, never rational when it comes to many basic choices. In one famous experiment, Flood offered individuals the choice between getting a $10 prize immediately versus a $15 prize if they could reach agreement with another person to give them any part, no matter how small, of the prize. The participants invariably chose immediate sure gain over future greater gain. Similar experiments have been repeated with similar results. People of all IQ levels overvalue immediate pleasures.

Money questions are far easier to make decisions about than selecting which foods to eat and when, since food offers immediate sensory pleasures; it is much harder to make rational choices with tasty temptations. So it is not snake oil food manufacturers or evil fast-food chains that make us fat. We do it to ourselves. Faced with the choice of potato chips now versus waiting for dinner in an hour or two, hungry people will take the chips now.

The healthy option, the option the individual *should* take, is sometimes taken, but not by many. Most of us suffer from what the Greeks called *akrasia*, or lack of self-control. When tasty food is plentiful and cheap and ubiquitous, we will eat more of it – unless a smart policy can outsmart us.

Government policy cannot easily overcome human desire. Yet a 2009 working group of U.S. regulatory agencies, including the Federal Trade Commission, believes it can.[134] In response to concerns about childhood obesity, they want to restrict the marketing of foods and beverages that contain significant amounts of sugar, sodium, and saturated fat. But the recommendations aren't binding; they act by what economists call 'moral suasion.' This group would also add a layer of bureaucracy to interpret the standards and provide guidance to advertisers. Similarly, in the UK, a 2009 Food Standards Agency report recommended that supermarkets sell skim milk and low-fat ice cream and cheese to help reduce saturated fats. Manufacturers would need to 'reformulate' their products, using less pastry in pork pies, for instance. According to Julian Hunt of the country's Food and Drink Federation, this policy recommendation doesn't stand a chance: 'Not one of our members ever receives a single complaint if they increase the size of their portions. But if they take out so much as one gram from a product, they are inundated with complaints.'[135]

Denial

Despite being armed with good information on how to eat right and exercise, adults fail to look after their own health. Furthermore, they fail to do it for their children. Amazingly, despite the obesity epidemic in America, Americans think they're in superb physical condition. Nearly 62 per cent of U.S. adults said they were in excellent or very good health, along with 82 per cent of their children, according to families sampled by the federal government for the National Health Interview Survey, conducted in 2007 and released in 2009.[136] When most parents don't acknowledge that their children are too fat, public health obesity prevention campaigns are clearly not hitting the mark. One might describe them as a complete waste of scarce resources.

Guidelines, subtle shaming tactics, and carpet-bombing social marketing get visibility and media attention. That's because they immediately demonstrate that the government is 'doing something,' even when the evidence, if soberly examined, is that these approaches do nothing of value to constrain the obesity epidemic. Even when shame is not involved – that is, even when plain cold facts are issued about public health safety – marketing campaigns are of questionable value. In the Province of Ontario, whose population of around 14 million is highly educated, just 37 per cent chose to get inoculated during the autumn of 2009 against the h1n1 flu virus – despite tens of millions of dollars spent by the provincial and federal governments on freestanding posters, on interior bus, subway, and train car ads in dozens of communities, on hundreds of newspapers ads (including multilingual ads), and on social media such as blogs and Facebook. Part of the problem with social marketing generally is the fragmentation of media. Just fifteen years ago, public health officials could channel communications through the major cable TV stations and newspapers and be certain they would capture a majority of the public. However, if many of your state's Chinese-born citizens read China-based websites, rather than local newspapers, you're going to have a harder, more expensive time reaching your target audiences.

Marketing messages may appeal to the public health industry because it's seen as retaliation against aggressive corporate ads for sugary cereals aimed at children. Yet public health ads cannot win this war against industry. Health officials are not 'selling' what people want to hear, so the public simply tunes out. Tired of being on the losing side of a head-to-head messaging war, public health marketers may be tempted to play to a base emotion, shame. This is not to suggest that some of the non–shame-based public health messages, if implemented, would not be effective; rather, it is to say that all these healthy-eating-and-exercise messages are not being absorbed, nor will they *ever* be absorbed, by those who need to pay them heed.

To be precise, the fault does sometimes lie in the message – it can be complex and contradictory. In one recent UK government anti-obesity campaign, funded at millions of taxpayer dollars, a primitive man is shown evolving from a hunter-gatherer to a couch potato lounging in front of the television. The message is unclear. Some viewers might see television watching as the peak of evolution, something to be emulated. Or they might perceive the message to be, 'Go back to hunting.' An editorial in *The Lancet*, the esteemed British medical journal, called the ad ridiculous and a waste of scarce public funds.

Or take the message of five servings of fruit and vegetables a day ('5 a day for better health' in California) – simple enough and certainly wholesome, but ultimately confusing when one also reads that this diet, by countering obesity, prevents stroke and bone loss but does nothing to stop breast cancer, which is also associated with obesity.[137] It's an amazingly complex world out there when it comes to obesity; simple weight loss messages that apply to everyone are hard to craft. The only way that health messaging can work is to have the person in the room with you and engage him in thoughtful discussion that explains personal risk carefully and sensitively. Risk is a very tricky subject for many of us to grasp, no matter how much higher education we've had. It's easy to hoodwink people. Many North Americans, for example, consider the label '100 per cent natural' to mean that it's healthy, but natural products (salt, for example) are not always healthy, especially not when the dose is high. Despite its popularity, the U.S. Food and Drug Administration has not established a clear definition for the term 'natural.'

Still, the fault more often lies, not with the ambiguous message, but with the fact that the healthful message is not absorbed. Poster campaigns to promote exercise may in fact make people eat more. In the study referred to earlier by Dolores Albarracin and her colleagues, college students were also asked to judge a series of posters from an exercise campaign; on another occasion, they were asked to judge a group of similar-looking posters that did not mention exercise. They were told they would be given a few raisins afterward, which they were to taste and rate. After the students examined the exercise posters, they ate an average of eighteen calories in raisins, but they ate only twelve calories after looking at the posters that did not mention exercise. Albarracin, the study's lead author, explained to the media that context was critical. 'When the setting of the advertising is more conducive to eating than exercise, people eat.' But as we've been stressing throughout this book, contexts vary with the individual. Each beholder looks through a very different eye.

A personalized approach to public health obesity policy should help each individual absorb the message in her own way and at her own pace and should eliminate the shame that attaches to traditional models of social messaging campaigns. Posters, pamphlets, informational websites, and subway campaigns carry little demonstrable benefit. Despite this, public health officials are tightening their embrace of them. In New York City, where half the population is overweight, city officials have launched a campaign in the subways reminding people that, for most adults, two thousand calories a day should be enough. Two problems here: subway commuters as a group are far slimmer than car commuters, and more important, the number 'two thousand' is meaningless to most people. Studies show that people are clueless as to how many calories they should consume in a day to maintain their current weight. The vast majority of people know that lots of calories mean a bigger bulge, but they don't process this rationally. Instead, many internalize it in such a way that they feel awful when they overeat and therefore eat more. Generic 'messaging' is not the answer, yet the popularity of this approach to fighting obesity is on the rise. Shame campaigns are the default public health communications programs these days, laced with unsubtle reminders that the obese are a disgrace.

Old Habits Die Hard

Despite consistently good intentions, public health has a mixed legacy when it comes to messaging campaigns. Take the case of hostile warning messages to those living in fear of AIDS – notably homosexual men during the 1980s. Early ads to prevent AIDS had the precisely opposite effect to what was intended. The evidence suggests that when they were made to feel more susceptible to the HIV virus than they in fact were, gay men tended to use condoms less often and, out of bravado, to be extra-promiscuous. The tens of millions spent on generic social marketing messages ('save your life; wear a condom') backfired.

Aggressive state marketing of the 'condom code' – that is, promoting the condom as a fail-safe means to prevent infection, while simultaneously condoning through law the supposedly liberating effects of anonymous gay sex in bathhouses – has been credited with speeding up the 'second wave' of AIDS in inner-city New York and San Francisco. Part of the problem was that, in the context of group sex, condoms need to be changed before every new sexual act. This message did not get through. It was anti-retroviral drugs and high-touch counselling through one-on-one support that turned AIDS into the less lethal, more manageable chronic condition that it is today in the Western world. Though one must be fair to condom messages: they did start to gain social traction once they were personally adopted by communities with which individuals self-identified – for example, gay, bisexual, drug-using, swinger communities.

Messages are perceived as shaming when they come from outsider groups, such as governments, that try to impose standards on individuals who have had nothing to do with establishing those standards. Gay groups reversed the shame by 'owning' the problem. Yet it is hard for the obese – a patchwork of disconnected sufferers – to own the problem, because social stigma has driven them into isolation, with each person who suffers from obesity suffering alone. Even though obesity is a health problem that strikes so many of us, there are few fancy fund-raising galas or well-heeled lobby groups representing the obese.

In the battle to control obesity, the results thus far from government public health messages have been depressing. Beginning in California, public health groups, the produce industry, and supermarkets rallied together to promote the health message of five servings of fruit and vegetables a day. By 1991 the California '5 A Day Program' had spanned the entire nation. Before launching the program, researchers ran a baseline survey to assess current intake, knowledge, and attitudes regarding fruit and vegetables. The survey found that U.S. adults were consuming 3.4 servings per day of fruit and vegetables and that less than one-quarter of Americans consumed fruit and vegetables five or more times per day.

Fifteen years later, Americans were eating far fewer fruits and vegetables despite a nationwide government-sponsored campaign to increase consumption. Yet they reported that they had 'heard' the message; a survey conducted in 1997 showed a significant increase in awareness of the '5 A Day' message. People, it seems, register the message cognitively, but something about the government telling them to eat their fruit and veggies just doesn't cut it. As Euripides famously said: 'Authority is never without hate.' People rebel. Or perhaps they don't know what a 'serving' is. More likely, as Martin Lindstrom has noted in the advertising and marketing context, people don't make purchasing decisions rationally when emotion guides decisions. And as we believe, emotion guides all food decisions at the point of purchase and at the point of consumption.

Governments – and people whom public health experts like to call anti-obesity 'champions' – persist in evangelizing fruits and veggies. 'Veggies taste so good when they come fresh from the garden, don't they?' Michelle Obama told a flock of children gathered around a soil tray on the fortieth anniversary of *Sesame Street*. 'If you eat all these healthy foods, you are going to grow up to be big and strong,' she smiles, flexing her fists. 'Just like me.'

Mrs Obama encourages parents to be better role models for their children. She has said that the epidemic of childhood obesity in America is 'eminently solvable' using the bully pulpit of the White House, plus fashionable big-state solutions: labelling laws and nutritious school breakfasts and lunches paid for by the taxpayer. She wants to promote physical education in schools and to broaden the appeal of walking and biking. She wants to stop marketing unhealthy chips and soda pop to children, enlisting the help of cartoon characters. A government report she commissioned called for food media companies to license popular cartoon characters only to healthy foods and beverages. It went on to threaten federal regulation of children's advertising if voluntary efforts failed. Weirdly, at the same time, after the release of her 120-page report in May 2010, she told reporters: 'Not a single expert that we've consulted has said that having the federal government tell people what to do is the way to solve this.' Yet new dietary guidelines from the Departments of Agriculture and Health and Human Services, released in 2010, in sync with her report, do exactly this. The guidelines, as they always do, preach that ever fatter

Americans should eat less fat, sugar, and salt and more vegetables and whole grains. But in addition to asking Americans to eat more healthfully, the Obama recommendations encourage adopting 'a more plant-based diet that emphasizes vegetables, cooked dry beans and peas, fruits, whole grains, nuts, and seeds.' Whatever her personal charisma, America has been down the Michelle Obama policy road many, many times before and come to a dead end. So called 'food labels,' the most vigorously supported of her policy proposals, are generally innocuous statements about portion size or packaging. Perhaps they're too innocuous. Foods can't claim that they are avenues toward better health, since this would require regulatory approval (such as by the FDA in the United States).

That's in part why claims around the superior health benefits of certain foods have to be generic and come from the state, not from the manufacturer ('eat five or more servings of fruits and vegetables'). This policy has been upheld in major U.S. court cases, notably *Pearson* v. *Shalala* (1999), in which the DC Court of Appeals precluded the FDA from marketing the health benefits of foods.[138] In 2003 the FDA allowed qualified health claims to appear on food labels as long as manufacturers' disclaimers noted the unreliability of the scientific connection between consuming the food and better health. But the 2003 FDA rule has been abandoned because the agency thought it was too confusing for consumers. So now the state is more in the driver's seat than ever when it comes to 'educating' and messaging to the public about what's healthy and what's not.

The most recent information on fruit and vegetable consumption in the United States is astounding in the degree to which it reveals the futility of the bully pulpit model.[139] Over the past eighteen years the percentage of U.S. adults aged forty to seventy-four eating five or more fruits and vegetables a day has decreased steadily. And those individuals for whom it matters most – those with a history of hypertension, diabetes, or cardiovascular disease – are no more likely to adhere to a healthy lifestyle than people without these conditions.

How do public health advocates and researchers interpret the lack of impact of the 5 A Day message? There wasn't *enough* money, they suggest. As the lobby group Consumers Union accurately noted in a press release, 'the ad budget for the top-spending fast food restaurants alone came in at $2.3 billion [in 2005], roughly 240 times greater than the communications budget for [all] the 5 A Day campaigns combined.'[140] What would have been enough money? The analysis by Consumers Union should suggest to policy makers that trying to match the competing power of the food industry is a waste of valuable resources.

Strangely, the U.S. 5 A Day initiative is held up by bureaucrats around the world as a success; in Canada, a report by the Chief Medical Officer for Ontario prodded the federal government to 'fund a national fruit and vegetable promotional campaign similar to the US 5 A Day to Better Health' program. In the fall of 2007, UK Department of Health officials said it would use simple messages – such as the 'five pieces of fruit and veg a day' slogan. 'Tackling obesity is the most significant public and personal health challenge facing our society,' said Health Secretary Alan Johnson as he launched the UK's £372 million strategy ('Change4Life').[141] Despite this, British eating habits and physical activity levels have deteriorated since the 2007 declaration. The number of British patients treated in hospital for obesity more than tripled from 2005 to 2009, with obesity-related admissions climbing by 60 per cent in 2009.

Mark Twain's understanding of the definition of insanity well describes the *modus operandi* of anti-obesity public health crusades throughout the Western world today: 'do the same thing again and again and hope for a different result.' Convincing people to eat their fruits and veggies may generate jobs in government public health offices, but it does little to advance the cause of obesity prevention. The motto of the Johns Hopkins Bloomberg School of Public Health champions 'protecting health, saving lives – millions at a time.' But if public health really is about protecting the 'millions,' it is surprising to learn that today's media campaigns to increase vegetable consumption – under way in every region across North America, and in much of Europe – show no evidence of return on investment. The Centers for Disease Control, which funds a great deal of the research in U.S. Schools of Public Health, admitted as much in 2009. When it published its first laundry list of large-scale community obesity prevention strategies in 2009, it said that data on effectiveness were scant. Said the CDC's Laura Kettel Khan: 'The whole concept of environmental and policy changes for obesity prevention is relatively new, so the evidence base is not very deep.'[142]

What Is 'Obesity Policy' Today?

What exactly do we mean by government 'policy' on obesity? What are governments saying and doing today about obesity? It's a colourful mix of blame-and-shame-and-mass-message policies, a pot-pourri of policy based on the axiomatic assumption that we are all the same – lemmings prepared to obey the dictates and clever messaging tactics of state health bureaucrats. It is arguably not really 'policy' at all. We reviewed government and public–private sector press releases on obesity prevention as announced during 2008. Here's some of what we found:

No Birthday Cakes Please!
WELLINGTON (Reuters) – Children have been banned from bringing cakes to share on their birthdays at a New Zealand school that is trying to clamp down on rising rates of childhood obesity.

Weight Limit Eases the Load on Beach Donkeys
Reuters News, 4 April 2008 – Relief is in sight for Britain's hard-working beach donkeys – from now on they won't have to carry anyone weighing more than eight stone (51 kg or 112 lb).

Love Your Veggies
OAKLAND, Calif., April 30 /PRNewswire/ – Actress and mother Kimberly Williams-Paisley wants kids everywhere to eat their veggies. *Henry and the Hidden Veggie Garden*, Williams-Paisley's first book, was written in support of the Love Your Veggies™ Nationwide School Lunch Campaign which today awarded 51 elementary schools each with a $10,000 nutrition grant.

UK Will Teach Kids to Cook to Fight Child Obesity
LONDON, Jan 22 (Reuters) – Cookery classes will be made compulsory in British secondary schools for the first time, the government announced on Tuesday, as the fight against childhood obesity intensifies.

Banning Junk Food Ads Targeting Children
TORONTO (Canadian Press) – Ontario is facing a 'serious problem' with overweight children and must do more to protect them by banning advertising directed at kids, NDP critic Rosario Marchese said. He plans to introduce a bill Monday amending the Consumer Protection Act to prohibit commercial television advertising for food or drink that is directed at a child under the age of 13. 'We believe that marketers know when marketing works and it does affect dietary choices that children make,' he said. 'We know that corporations hire a lot of psychologists to market

adequately to every category of age groups that one can think of. So we know that it affects kids.'

Parents of Obese Children May Get Warning Letters
LONDON, Oct 22 (Reuters) – Parents of severely overweight children could be sent letters warning them of the health dangers involved, the government said on Monday.

New Regulatory Regime to Prevent Marketing Junk Food to Children
OTTAWA, March 5 /CNW Telbec/ – A panel of prominent, independ-ently minded Canadians ranging from educators, Aboriginal, community and youth leaders, journalists, public policy researchers, academics and authors, today released a recommendation for a made in Canada plan to ensure that unhealthy food and beverages are not marketed to children.

Based on our summary of press releases from the major U.S. and Canadian newswires, we synthesized the four most popular currently emerging policy approaches to the problem of obesity across the indus-trialized world.

1. *Policies that champion incentives to change behaviour.* The cen-trepiece of this strategy, of which there are many subvarieties, is insur-ance reform to reduce what economists call 'moral hazard' – the idea that people will overuse insured services if overuse carries no negative consequence. The flip side of this policy coin is to introduce a 'Pegouvi-an'-style tax – that is, a sin or welfare tax – to tax the externalities (costs) of weight gain.

Taxation can be a highly effective tool to motivate behaviour change: as cigarette taxes go up, consumption generally falls, especially because potential new users consider the habit too expensive to start and give it a miss. Consider that one can of regular soda has the equivalent of ten teaspoons of sugar – leading, eventually, to billions of dollars in medi-cal costs. A health tax on the soda could, in theory, punish the manu-facturer and the supplier (that is, the sugar industry). This approach, most germane to a public payer model of health care (such as found in Canada or the United Kingdom), presupposes that obesity carries an external price, akin to environmental pollution, insofar as the obese impose costs on the taxpayer by overloading emergency wards and by burdening the health care system.

Estimates are that over a lifetime, the typical Type 2 diabetes patient in a public payer model costs the state about three times as much as a non-diabetic in terms of direct medical and hospitalization costs. According to the Center for Science in the Public Interest, for every penny of tax added to a twelve-ounce bottle of soda, consumption of all those empty calories would drop by 1 per cent. The problem is one of fairness in the design of any such tax: How are we to ensure that it does not unduly hurt the poor (which it certainly would do)? And how are we to select which industries should be punished – non-diet sodas only? What about corn syrup manufacturers? Avocado producers?

Former New York Governor David Paterson proposed an 18 per cent tax on sugary drinks but abandoned the idea after lobbyists correctly pointed out that such a tax would land unfairly on lower-income families.[143] In poor areas beset by high rates of obesity (such as East Harlem), the soda tax would have zero impact on consumers' decisions since soda is cheap and plentiful; it would be a sin tax that benefited only the university-educated upper-middle class – the ones most in favour of the idea. The motive behind the tax was to raise $400 million a year, modelled after the notion of the cigarette tax, which has been credited with saving 40,000 lives per year (based on teenagers whom you've stopped from taking up the habit). The critical difference, however, between a soda pop tax and a tobacco tax is the 'exhaustiveness principle.' There aren't many tobacco substitutes, so the tax captures the market, whereas a soda pop tax would simply push up demand for non-pop sugary and caloric substitutes. Also, the legal costs (borne by the taxpayer) in fighting such a tax in the courts would be massive. The cola industry would justifiably scream commercial discrimination. As Kevin Keane, the industry association's spokesman said in 2008: 'If you're serious about obesity, you're not going to make a dent in it by singling out one product.'[144]

Besides, most economists generally don't like taxes as a way to cut down on obesity. It's much too blunt an instrument. A tax on food is unlikely to reduce obesity by much unless it is set very high, and while such a tax might ultimately help those who are obese, it would penalize the majority – those who aren't obese. After all, food is a necessity of life, unlike cigarettes.

2. *Policies that educate and badger people into taking weight control seriously.* In none of these social marketing or government 'persuasion' initiatives – in the form of public service ads on buses and subways and in schools – are the outcomes evidence based. That is, there has never been a single study anywhere as far as we are aware that uses what epidemiologists call a randomized control trial, with longitudinal data

(that is, evaluations over time) tracking two separate groups, one subject to a social marketing campaign and one not, to show whether badgering people to lose weight in fact works. These campaigns are usually based on 'best practices' developed by small, consensus-based panels of public health academics or public relations and communications specialists. The panel of supposed experts announced by the Canadian federal government, in the press release presented earlier ('New Regulatory Regime to Prevent Marketing Junk Food to Children'), is one such example. The moderator of this state-funded 'consensus panel' was Avi Lewis, a prominent member of Canada's left-leaning establishment, which is partial to state-sponsored activities. At times, these policies are aimed at parents of infants or children, in recognition of the family-based nature of weight problems and their solutions. At times, they are targeted to groups at risk (new moms, recent immigrants, Aboriginals). Generally, however, they are what we call 'carpet-bombing' message campaigns, since it costs enormous sums to adjust social marketing campaigns to the sensitivities of specific groups. Even within groups, people's reactions to a campaign of this sort are unpredictable.

In the case of cigarettes, graphic warning labels of lungs (shot through with thick holes) placed on cigarette packages are the most celebrated of such messaging initiatives, but there is very little evidence that even those worked as they were intended. Many individuals stop going to anti-smoking classes precisely because they are so offended by the graphics. In the best-known 'neuromarketing studies,' which look at the effects of marketing on the smoker's brain using functional magnetic resonance imaging (fMRI), researchers found that dire anti-smoking messages (Portuguese packs stating that 'Smoking Kills') swelled the *nucleus accumbens*, the brain's so-called craving spot. As with smokers, the obese may feel badly shamed when confronted with not so subtle generic anti-obesity or healthy eating images, but this in no way makes them want to snack less. It may do the very opposite.

3. *Policies that impose greater regulation on industry to promote healthy choices.* These initiatives have so far been totally ineffective. The public's desire for fatty, high-sodium, high-calorie foods is too strong. The prices of fruits and vegetables are climbing faster than inflation throughout the industrialized world, while junk food is everywhere becoming much, much cheaper and more accessible. Meanwhile, the heavy-regulation approach rubs up against the incessant drum roll of public health messages that exhort us to take individual responsibility ('The power of willpower!'). This sends conflicting signals to the pub-

lic. Regulatory taxes attach to the manufacturer, not to the individual; as such, those taxes hit the bottom lines of the junk food producers. If the policy is not designed effectively, manufacturers can of course pass on the costs of those taxes to the consumer. Some anti-obesity campaigns have been less antagonistic to industry and have worked to convince grocery chains, restaurants, and associations that they can win market share if they introduce healthy options. Many in the public health academic community feel this is just a sham to fight off government regulation by creating the appearance of voluntary changes. Whatever the motive, the policy has proven itself a dismal health failure everywhere it has been tried. When McDonald's introduced more healthy options, healthier people came, but the obese still bought the Big Macs and cinnamon buns. This is good public relations for McDonald's, but bad public policy if governments were to force such change on food industry chains. For a decade, food companies have liked to say they have been working 'with government' to reduce high-caloric options. In the summer of 2010, sixteen major U.S. food makers promised to cut 1.5 trillion calories from their products by 2015 to support the First Lady's White House campaign to combat obesity. Yet it will be impossible to tell whether anyone's cooperating, unless public health officials investigate activities at the food plants.

The futility of these policy approaches having been recognized, the latest avenue for fighting industry has been in the courts.[145] Class action lawsuits, especially in the United States, are quickly putting the fast-food industry on the defensive. At the same time, human rights lawyers are gearing up to combat a rising number of discrimination claims launched by the obese (relating, for example, to higher prices for airline and movie tickets). The obese are increasingly suing doctors for failing to properly advise them as to the health risks of weight gain. This in itself suggests that the 'trusted' relationship between doctor and patient has frayed badly and that we have a far way to go in promoting a culture of meaningful doctor–patient dialogue about obesity control.

The biggest court battle in the human rights context hit the news in 2008, when Canada's Supreme Court ruled that fat people are entitled to two seats on an airplane for the price of one. News of the ruling reverberated throughout the international media, for in effect it declared obesity to be a disability; thus, obese airline passengers were entitled to human rights protections in the same way as, say, wheelchair-bound passengers.

Air Canada and WestJet, another Canadian airline, had sought to overturn the 'one person, one fare' policy enacted by the Canadian Transportation Agency in January 2007. Here's how Paul McAleer, the former 'fat acceptance' activist and past editor of bigfatblog.com – a leading fat acceptance blog between 2000 and 2008 – initially reacted to the 2007 Agency decision: 'All in all, this is a superb ruling and the Canadian Transportation Agency should be applauded for upholding our rights, enforcing their ruling, and allowing fat people to fly with dignity – something that the loudmouthed "thin" people on the internet are taking for granted.'

We should note here that while complainant Linda McKay-Panos was overjoyed by her victory in the agency ruling, the airline industry is still fuming over it and figuring out ways to circumvent it. Warren Everson, spokesman for the Air Transportation Association of Canada, told CBC's *Marketplace:* 'If the government of Canada feels that people who are overweight need special societal benefit, then the government should provide it, not put it on the backs of shareholders and other customers.'

4. *The medical response.* New surgical devices and fashionable drug remedies such as Lipitor™ are delaying the costs of obesity, potentially putting off the heart disease, cancers, and other ills wrought by poor eating behaviour. Some natural experiments *have* indicated that bariatric surgery performed on severely obese teenagers may be more long-lasting and cost effective than all other forms of weight control aimed at those who are young and obese. Very recent research has found that obese teens randomly assigned to receive weight loss surgery dropped significantly more weight than obese teenagers randomly selected to pursue the 'Michelle Obama' prescription for weight loss – that is, a reduced-calorie diet and exercise. Many surgeons and other medical practitioners – some of whom are disdainful of public health government workers and simple public health marketing – favour this approach, though surgery is only for the *very* obese. Unlike the other common policy responses to obesity management and prevention discussed so far, the medical approach is not overtly shaming. It treats obesity like any other disease. Yet by viewing obesity as a classifiable disease, as opposed to a *risk factor* for disease, it can be seen as stigmatizing in the same sense that 'premenstrual syndrome' as a diagnosis is considered stigmatizing of women; and 'homosexuality' as a psychiatric label was considered (until it was officially removed from the psychiatric diagnostic manual) potentially stigmatizing by the gay and lesbian community.

The very process of diagnosis differentiates a person from others and is, therefore, potentially humiliating, especially when the person is already feeling vulnerable. All labels eventually degenerate into pejorative terms. If, as we believe, the vast majority of people are confronted with challenges of weight management or are at risk of being so confronted, then we need to craft a public policy approach that sees *all* people as being at risk for obesity (though each in individual ways), instead of designing such policies to 'conquer' obesity, as if it were cancer or diabetes or a more easily classifiable disease.

Based on our review, most recent government announcements in the realm of obesity policy celebrate option 2: social marketing or moral suasion. Why so? Social mass marketing is cheapest and politically the most saleable. Data that we present in chapter 4 indicate high levels of public support for government anti-obesity marketing policies that tell people to keep fit and eat right. The odd thing about this is that the proof for such policies is not in any pudding we know. Scouring the academic literature, it's difficult to find more than a handful of social marketing or message campaigns where the message itself – whether it's 5 A Day in California or 'Stay Active Stay Independent' in New South Wales – enjoys significant and lasting recognition beyond Year One; in other words, people may not distinguish the campaign for physical activity and healthy living from Viagra endorsements. They push the same mute button for both. They are on autopilot, or on their BlackBerries, and they just don't care.

Whatever the policy approach, different top-down anti-obesity initiatives we have reviewed here have very different strategic goals. These goals can be divided into three basic categories: first, promoting healthy behaviours (such as eating your vegetables and spending time in the park) – which, even if successful, may not actually do anything to reduce weight; second, reducing weight (a much more ambitious goal); or third, preventing weight gain (a long-term strategy usually targeted at children under six). There is inevitably overlap among goals.

Of the three, promoting healthy behaviours is, from a social marketing perspective, the easiest approach to sell politically. The problem – the eight-hundred-pound gorilla in the policy world of the public health establishment – is that there is no compelling evidence that sending out broad messages about healthy behaviour reduces weight at all. In fact, the very lack of correlation between healthy behaviour (for example, eating from among a rich variety of food groups) and weight loss is frustrating: you follow the rules and nothing happens. So you run to the fridge for solace.

Of course, we're not *against* funding public schools to make fresh fruit, vegetables, and low-fat milk freely available to schoolchildren. This may provide some children with the nutrients they need for learning. We support summer camps that emphasize good nutrition and exercise. We agree that the public should be warned about the dangers of starvation diets. And we think that seriously overweight people should have the same legal protections and benefits offered to people with comparable disabilities. But the issue in this book is what policy might best work to combat obesity. What policy option delivers the most return on investment? In the West, policy makers are all flummoxed by the colossal cost problems of obesity. No public policies so far seem to have made an appreciable dent. So we support trying something new, something that might actually work in a sustained way, something that encourages real change.

4 Healthy Living Vouchers

Content makes poor men rich; discontent makes rich men poor.

Benjamin Franklin

Lessons from School Choice

What makes the poor content? What makes social disadvantage fade? We believe the answer lies in equal opportunity, be it in education or in personal health. One of the most powerful and promising policies to improve school scores for the poor in the U.S. and elsewhere has been the introduction of 'school choice.' It is a policy of emancipation.

School choice is a term used to describe programs that give families the opportunity to choose the school they want their children to attend. Their options are public schools within or outside their residential area, private schools, charter schools, or home schooling (with the aid of tax credits or vouchers). School choice is a policy once linked to the free market wing of the U.S. Republican Party. Yet today it enjoys its strongest political support among traditionally Democratic black voters on the poverty line. In politics, this is referred to as a 'wedge issue': people vote with their hearts and feet, not their party affiliation. Referendums coinciding with U.S. congressional elections indicate that African Americans have generally been highly supportive of school choice policy.[146]

Poor African American families in inner-city Baltimore, Chicago, Washington, and Milwaukee love the concept of being able to enrol their children in private schools because it provides them with hope for a better future for their children. They also favour charter schools –

public elementary and secondary schools that receive public money but enjoy some autonomy in curriculum in exchange for more accountability in terms of results, such as high graduation rates. This is why the Bill and Melinda Gates Foundation, which focuses on elevating the hopes of the poor around the world, has given millions of dollars in support of charter schools in heavily black cities such as Houston. Today there are more charter schools per capita in Harlem than anywhere in America. Harlem charter students are outscoring their white peers in suburbia. In 2010, Harlem's charter schools had more than eleven thousand applicants for two thousand slots. Why are the poor so excited by the choice that charter schools offer them?

The poor have been stagnating in regulated neighbourhood public schools – quagmires of lost opportunity. America has thousands of high schools, and a mere 10 per cent of them produce half of all dropouts. A black child in America has a 50 per cent chance of attending one of these failing schools. Parents want what is best for their children, and they know their own children better than state bureaucrats do. Martin Luther King Jr insisted that the answer to solving America's race problem was improving the quality of schools for all children. Even today, with a black president in the White House, fewer than half of America's African American students (but 89 per cent of white students) attend high schools where graduation is the norm. The poor are like all other parents – they want what is best for their children; they know what is best for their children – but they differ in that they have much more to lose if their children drop out of school. Freedom of choice to attend the school in one's state that best fits a child's need – a fit that offers real hope of emancipation from poverty – should, we feel, be considered a basic human right.

Milton Friedman, winner of the Nobel Prize for Economics in 1976, saw hopelessness writ large on the faces of children in inner-city public schools across America. It prompted him to ask tough questions about the state monopoly in public education. He believed that the poor had reason to revolt, and he conceived the idea of educational vouchers as the best way for individuals to guarantee challenge and opportunity for their children. Vouchers would vastly increase the variety of schools that children could choose to attend, so he promoted niche schools, from the arts to dance, to religion-based curricula, to science, to mathematics, to civics. Schools could compete for vouchers, improving their standards as they competed. They could get rid of bad ideas, improve on good ideas, and vie for top spot in their respective niches.

Friedman, as any student of economics knows well, was one of the twentieth century's greatest proponents of the 'invisible hand' of market forces. The 'invisible hand' was economist Adam Smith's now legendary metaphor for the confluence of self-interest, competition, and supply and demand that drove the entirety of economic exchange. Vouchers, believed Friedman, would allow government 'to serve its proper function of improving the operation of the invisible hand without substituting the dead hand of bureaucracy.'[147]

Today we know that school choice vouchers have improved grades in low-income families for tens of thousands of school-age children across North America. Roughly three-quarters of low-income families who received educational vouchers for private schools across Canada have rated their educational experience as an 'A.'[148] Educational vouchers have improved reading, writing, and mathematics scores among low-income, inner-city African American children.[149] In New York and Chicago, poor black students in charter schools outperform their more affluent counterparts. In Milwaukee, voucher students in the Parental Choice Program between 2003 and 2008 enjoyed a substantially greater graduation rate than kids in local public schools.

Yet it is recognized, even among ardent supporters of school vouchers, that it can take decades for broader, sustained benefits to roll in, in the form of higher college graduation rates, steady employment, rising incomes and accomplishments, a stable family life, and so on. Groundswell support among the poor for education vouchers makes sense: they want to be poor no longer, and they aspire to equality and opportunity. Poor in material goods but wealthy in ambition for their children, they want to escape the ghetto, and the best way out is through education.

Another way out of a grim future is through better health.

Vouchers and Obesity

Would the poor embrace 'healthy living' vouchers in the same way they embrace education vouchers? Do the same rules of human motivation apply? Imagine giving real cash, and therefore real choice, to help people live healthier lives. Imagine ending the monopoly in setting obesity policy via state-knows-best educational campaigns. Imagine offering *individuals* the chance to solve the greatest public health challenge of the twenty-first century: obesity.

Poor families have few choices when it comes to opportunities for healthy living and eating. The urban poor are surrounded by liquor stores and fast-food outlets, not fresh fruit stores. A fundamental need – the need for health, free from obesity-related illness – is not being met. This is especially so for the poor and disenfranchised in America's inner cities. They are generally heavier than their better-off peers and their diets are higher in fried food and salt content.

Tracy Parson, a Toronto mother on government social assistance whose children benefited from educational vouchers, says that vouchers to subsidize gym memberships, athletic team memberships, or the purchase of groceries – or any number of other options that she and her neighbours could immediately use – would be just as helpful to her family as educational vouchers have been. Many poor families would love to provide their children with tailored weight management opportunities but are unable to do so due to financial constraints, she says. Vouchers offer a buffet of options for poor people who struggle with their weight.

Educational school-choice vouchers allowed Ms Parson to send her children to a school more sensitive to her son's learning disability. Obesity vouchers, or what we call 'healthy living vouchers' (HLVs), would be similar in their sensitivity to a person's specific behavioural needs in weight loss and weight management. Special exercise stamps geared to specific needs, for both children and adults, would work, she believes, for obesity. So might special-use allowances for organic meats and dairy products at markets frequented by the rich or middle class, like Whole Foods.

Another mom on social assistance, Elisabeth Loduca, told us that educational vouchers and obesity vouchers are equally powerful in their promise: 'Obesity vouchers would be just as useful in everyday life because of the commitment you've made to better your life. This is what in my opinion the educational voucher has done for my children and for our family.'

Pastor Jeff Eastwood of Northside Baptist Church in Waterloo, Ontario, says that HLVs could substantially benefit his poor parishioners. Any type of financial help, he says, provides the freedom to make decisions that were not previously available: lack of resources over weight management, he believes, stops the discussion before it can even get started.

Behind any voucher scheme is a plan to offer people the basic right to pursue a range of options, be it in education or healthier living and eating. Before learning precisely how the lesson of educational vouchers might apply to obesity management, however, let's look more widely at experiments around the world that have tried to induce people to make healthier decisions.

When Do We Act to Better Our Health?

Behavioural economics, briefly introduced earlier in this book, is the study of when and why we change our behaviour in response to financial incentives. In health care there have been a number of small-scale experiments testing human behavioural responses to economic incentives, such as cash rewards to people who engage in activities to better their health.

There have, for example, been 'regret lotteries' – teams of people lose their bet if they fail to beat other teams in pre-defined health goals. Experiments have been undertaken with 'deposit contracts,' where people commit beforehand to a healthy behaviour by putting money down in advance. Some of these experiments appear to have led to slightly healthier behaviour in some people. Other experiments have resulted in little, if any, positive change, like the case of one Virginia doctor who gave his obese patients a dollar for every pound they shed.[150] It is difficult to distinguish truth from fiction regarding many of these experiments, since they have mostly come in the form of small-scale consulting studies for private sector organizations and have seldom been evaluated independently. Furthermore, all studies of which we are aware have involved small amounts of money, with the healthy options and potential 'winnings' defined by the experimenter, not by the test subject. For HLVs to work, as we shall argue, there needs to be a major financial inducement, and most important, the variety of healthy options needs to be extraordinarily diverse so that people, in collaboration with their health professional, can choose among them.

What we do know with certainty is that unhealthy individual choice drives the majority – roughly 70 per cent – of health care spending in most industrialized countries. And the majority of bad health choices that cause health care costs to rise involve people eating too much of the wrong thing too often. Furthermore, people of all ages and education levels are eating fewer and fewer fruits and vegetables and are increasingly sedentary. The one outlier category, described in chapter 3, is the megarich, who can afford the leisure time to exercise intensively and who are influenced by peer group norms of strict diet and heavy workout regimes. (They can probably also afford the occasional elective bariatric surgery, too.) This means that today, individuals' life choices determine an increasingly large proportion of medical burden and cost. If we could influence consumer behaviour for the better, we would improve health and the value of the money we invest in the prevention and cure of obesity-related chronic disease.

The central challenge is not simply to motivate; more fundamentally, it is to sustain healthy behaviour change. Short of making hamburgers and fries taste so awful that people won't buy them, this is hard work. Behavioural economics theory dresses down the assumption that all of us are purely rational agents. Consider this: there is no change in calories purchased after governments force restaurants to label food calories. How can this be? Here is the problem with the 'eat your fruits and vegetables' campaign mentality: when obese individuals are faced with a death sentence, *when they are literally told by a clinician in a public service announcement to expect an early death if they don't change their life-style immediately*, they still make little change over the long term. Some do, but most don't. If being told that they run the risk of death won't motivate most people to change their ways, why do we expect 'eat your veggies' campaigns to make a whit of difference?

As a society supposedly concerned about weight – maintaining a healthy weight for their children is a dominant concern of most young parents – we do not respond rationally to information alone, no matter how authoritative that information may sound. Most obese people do not consider themselves to be overweight. Information labels, even when backed up by stern warnings of the Grim Reaper, and even when delivered by confidence-inspiring, silver-haired doctors, accomplish little. *But,* and here's the take-home point, each of us is distinct in genetic, physiological, and psychological make-up, and each of us is irrational in a uniquely individual way. This is predictable and borne out. We therefore need to design intelligent weight loss and weight management solutions that take advantage, and celebrate, each individual's unique irrationality. Every individual has emotional biases that affect how he or she makes decisions about how to eat. Health professionals and policy makers need to heed these biases and advise accordingly.

Subsidize the Consumer: Our Policy Solution

Just as with education, the issue of obesity is one that consumers need to own in order to make meaningful change. Right now we pay our taxes so that public health bureaucrats can tell us to 'get moving' or 'eat right.' Does social marketing of this kind have a high return on investment? As we've noted already, the evidence defiantly tells us 'no.' Our policy solution is to stop subsidizing the current producer of anti-obesity sloganeering – the state, through its public health messaging and healthy eating campaigns – and to start subsidizing individuals so that they have more choice over how to curb their own obesity. In an interview on public education and government intervention, Milton Friedman made precisely the same point when discussing education: 'Subsidizing the producer is the wrong way to do it because it creates a top-down organization, which is very inefficient. The better way is to subsidize the consumer, which is what vouchers do.'[151]

As obvious as this next point may sound, it's important to note that ours is a *policy* response. It is not an advocacy response, which we hear a lot about, from, among others, the American Civil Liberties Union, the Center for Science in the Public Interest, and the National Association for Fat Acceptance. Nor is it a gold standard, purely evidence-based approach, because good policy cannot wait for research solutions to obesity. Research is never finite, especially in obesity, where, as we've seen, the results of studies are in eternal flux and rife with complexity, contradiction, and biospecific science (that is, with information of value to some and, therefore, valueless to others). Even the tool that researchers have been using to measure obesity – BMI – has been cast aside by many experts as unreliable. Finally, ours is a policy that loves liberty; some on the right and left of the political spectrum may dismiss our idea as 'libertarian paternalism.' Yes, we *do* encourage a kind of desired conduct – losing weight – by making it financially attractive to do so. But in just the same way that school choice advocates encourage children to get an excellent formative education, we want to do the same with healthy eating. And we do so by offering people meaningful choices about how to lose weight.

If you have ever fought with an expanding waistline, then you know the oft-touted culprits: too much food and too little exercise. Every teenager and adult knows this – but that information is meaningless when couched in bland marketing messages. And even *tailoring* the persuasion messages – telling, for example, geriatric women to 'get up and move slowly,' or telling new moms to 'exercise so that they can look good in a bathing suit if *they* want to' – has limited to no impact on individuals seeking to lose weight. Yes, the less you move (calories out) and the more you eat (calories in), the more fat you will accumulate. But as we have noted, researchers around the world are finding – with near daily media reports – increasingly relevant evidence of new twists to old information, new causes of obesity: fatty food 'addiction'; diet soda; the anti-inflammatory adipokine; the bacteria in your gut; DNA markers; sleep apnea; lack of brown fat cells; the hormone leptin; serotonin uptake rates; fibre intake rates; medications; depression; poverty; who your friends are; and so on. The growing universe of fat culprits and enablers is dizzying. All we really know now is that we don't know enough.

We believe that to change the cycle of futile social marketing campaigns in public health, and to treat people with dignity, respectful public policy – so often sidelined in the discussions around obesity – needs to be taken seriously. Politicians, as we've seen, tend to shy away from developing an official obesity policy. Why is this? We feel that this is partly due to anti-corporate animus.

There is almost universal medical acknowledgment that obesity is 'multipronged' – fashionable jargon in the modern obesity researcher's lexicon. But at the same time, there is no policy afoot anywhere in the world that relies heavily – or more than cosmetically – on private enterprise to combat obesity. Consider that in 2009, dozens of prominent doctors resigned proudly from the American Academy of Family Physicians after it accepted a grant from Coca-Cola to pay for education about the dietary role of beverages and sweeteners. A 2009 editorial in *The Lancet* lambasted the UK government for getting into bed with corporations to fight obesity:

> It beggars belief that the government has decided to allow sponsorship by commercial companies in the order of £200 million, in addition to £75 million of public funding ... Party to this sponsorship arrangement are also supermarkets that display rows upon rows of sugary snacks, cereals, and soft drinks.[152] The government justifies its decision by the need to tap into the power of brand loyalties, and the fact that these companies have influence with the target audience.

If obesity is, in fact, 'multipronged,' one would think that a multipronged strategy would want to *embrace* the intelligence and resources of industry. Yet much of the public health academic community considers the private sector evil; so much for the rhetoric of 'cross-sectoral linkages,' another popular term often tossed about by public health physicians and academic researchers. Scorning the private sector, governments prefer to cloak their anti-obesity or healthy living messages in the veil of 'public health promotion' – which is often nothing more than gently shaming the victim, with little or no effectiveness to show for it. We are not the only ones who have noted the lack of attention paid to serious obesity policy. Kelly Brownell, director of the Rudd Center for Food Policy and Obesity at Yale, notes that 'while there are a number of scientific groups dealing with obesity, they tend not to deal with public policy.'[153] Our aim is to nudge governments to take obesity policy seriously so as to make a difference for individuals. Even if our specific policy recommendation, HLVs, goes unheeded, we hope we can encourage a meaningful policy debate.

Like educational vouchers, HLVs could give individuals choice over how they can best take care of their bodies in order to slim down and keep fit, with government money going right to consumers to enable that choice. Individuals, working with their primary care providers, should know best what works for them ... *if* they are given a truly varied suite of options to consider and the financial means to take advantage of them.

We know from survey data around the world that, while individuals are influenced in their health decisions via many sources, including their family and friends, and including online friends whom they have never physically met, a primary care provider is the most influential source of health care information for any individual, and we suspect this will be the case for some time to come, even if that care provider's advice eventually reaches the patient through the Internet or iPhone or another remote electronic gadget. That is why the primary care provider would need to work hand in hand with the patient to make our policy work.

Many individuals, of course, don't know exactly why they have fallen into the overweight class or they wouldn't be in the predicament they're in. So primary health care providers need to be intensely involved in order to listen to their patients and advise them effectively. Those providers need to be well reimbursed for their thorough knowledge about healthy choices and for the time they spend recommending those choices, counselling patients, and guiding them in the right direction over the long haul. As we shall see, part of our policy recommendation is that primary care providers be given a strong, ongoing financial incentive in supporting HLV policies.

The technical mechanics of our proposed policy are important, but first let's remind ourselves why we need to move away from top-down government approaches. Prominent examples of this expensive top-down approach include the following: rolling out school district posters and websites and virally marketed videos that order us to lose weight and eat right; legislating that public school unions get into the swimming school business (through a mandatory daily offering to students); mandating school-wide minimum recess times; expanding urban green spaces; entrenching bike lanes in inner cities. The list goes on and on. But here's the problem with the top-down philosophy: there is no such thing as the 'average patient' or the 'average child' when it comes to obesity.

Imagine an academic paper in the music field enjoining parents to start music appreciation for their children by age three to bring out the musical abilities of each and every one. Imagine the state then advocating a policy solution: finance the 'Suzuki method' for all school-age children!

We do not have an opinion on the Suzuki method – which teaches youngsters to appreciate music before they can read – yet clearly, children are born with a wide range of musical abilities, and the Suzuki method may or may not be for them. Even Suzuki method junkies would find it absurd if the state were to force the approach on all children at taxpayers' expense. Every parent knows that even very musical children have unique windows of time during which they are more or less attuned to learning music. It would be wrong to treat all children with the same instructive method and at the same early age. So why do public health officials pursue this kind of 'sameness' logic when it comes to obesity?

Sameness logic explains the failure of multimillion-dollar megaphone campaigns to encourage the eating of fruits and vegetables for the masses as a means of effective weight control. Despite tens of millions of taxpayer dollars spent on this top-down policy, an October 2009 survey by Dietitians of Canada found that almost one-quarter of Canadians don't eat fruits or vegetables on a daily basis.[154] Good eating habits have deteriorated steadily in the past decade, though there has been a huge investment in public health education and badgering across the Western world. It hasn't worked because it has been aimed at the 'average' individual, a person who doesn't exist.

N of 1

In scientific terms, obesity, as we have learned, is what some thinkers, notably prominent patient advocates such as Jen S. McCabe, call an 'N of 1 problem.' She has designed a popular Web and mobile phone application that embraces the N of 1 philosophy. On the website imoveyou. com, every participant enters a 'commitment contract' with a person whom she trusts. She then commits to a simple exercise regimen she thinks will work for her. She barters with the other person; that is, if she fails, she loses money or something else of value to her.

An 'N of 1 problem' is a problem where the only sample size of statistical relevance is 1 (that is, an N of 1). When it comes to weight, everyone is physiologically and biochemically unique. It is well known that individuals do not respond in the same way to the same treatment. When taking identical doses of the same drug, some people fare well while others fall sick. Six to seven per cent of hospital admissions in the U.S. are due to idiosyncratic, adverse drug reactions from otherwise innocuous drugs. People are different. As obvious as this may sound, this observation is totally counter-intuitive to public health policy, public health research, and public health advocacy.

In traditional public health studies, a large sample size is seen as critical when evaluating the power of what researchers call 'interventions.' The greater the numbers of people (N) enrolled in the study, the better. If eating habits, *on average*, improve over time in the study arm that receives the anti-obesity intervention (say, time spent looking at anti–junk food posters on subways), obesity researchers will treat the finding as important.

Example of a Public Health Finding

To keep this example simple, we're exaggerating to make a point: Let's say there are ten people in a study of an obesity treatment. The program begins. During the study, one person gets sick with a rotten flu and loses thirty pounds as a result. By follow-up time, he's still thirty pounds down while eight of the others have neither gained nor lost, and one person has gained five pounds. So, altogether, this group lost twenty-five pounds over the study period. This means, on average, that each of the ten participants has lost 2.5 pounds and the treatment is pronounced a success! The results are published, and clinics around the country copy the treatment, trying to replicate the original findings. Of course, in real life, the sample size is much larger and fancy statistical regression models are used to weed out, or 'adjust for,' confounding factors (such as the flu and sex and age) that may have affected the outcome. But the point we're making is that it is *impossible* to capture all the confounders in the context of obesity. The researchers may not hear about them and so cannot possibly adjust for them. The other point is that, while some people may well lose weight (that is, the program is effective for them), the weight gain of the majority will obscure the success of the few. The group, when taken as a whole, will fail to show results, so that a treatment that works only for a few will go unnoticed. The control or untreated group may do just as well as the treated group for inexplicable reasons (the extra attention of being in a study may motivate them to diet). At the end, a mediocre intervention may seem to be great; an excellent intervention (for the tiny few) will never see the light of day.

There are lots of problems in trying to track the success of public health anti-obesity programs. We have to predict, notice, and document complex and often subtle intervening events (illness, pregnancy, death in the family, change in income) that will skew results. We have to keep track of all the potentially effective interventions at play (group support, rivalry, attention) and sort out who responded to what and why. Everything we now know about the genetics and psychology of obesity indicates that people will respond differently to different obesity programs. Complexity apart, 'on average,' outcomes from these big top-down programs – as with poor, inner-city school programs – are dismal, despite all the money we've invested so far.

Individualism vs Collectivism and the Impact of Vouchers

Yale psychologist Rebecca Puhl, among the most prominent and academically influential of obesity researchers in the world, believes that individualistic cultures in which people are uniquely responsible for themselves contribute to the widespread blame directed toward people with obesity.[155] Puhl points out that obese people in the UK and Australia are likely to be stigmatized because both these states are individualistic and believe in personal responsibility, unlike Venezuela, India, and Turkey, which are considered collectivist countries. We disagree – and have collected and analysed the data to prove it, as we will show later in this chapter. Industrialized and non-industrialized nations suffer alike from obesity (to differing degrees), though there may well be countries where the obese are more accepted and less derided than they are in America.

In a heavily collectivist culture, like Cuba, there may arguably be slightly more deference to authority to the point that 'megaphone' public health messages may indeed be relatively more effective. Culture is important in determining what makes us fat or thin. The effectiveness of programs increases when public health messages respect the traditions of those they address, for instance, traditional beliefs about harmony and balance (balancing cold with hot foods) – another example of the need to individualize the message. Our approach, HLVs, could still be used in collectivist cultures, but those vouchers would, perhaps, best be distributed to clan leaders or family patriarchs rather than to individuals because that's the way the culture works.

In North America, vouchers will work, we argue, precisely because of our individualistic inclinations. We take individualism seriously, for such is the nature of obesity and of the market society in which we live. We want to give individuals real power over how they can improve their weight, an intensely individual dilemma. We believe that all people want to be fit, but they need a better arsenal of resources and tools to make it happen. So our solution is this: let's literally give individuals the means to put where their mouth is. This approach, we call HLVs.

Vouchers: Some First Principles

To understand what we mean by HLVs, we will first return to the topic of educational vouchers, which stimulated this idea. The concept of vouchers grew out of the educational choice movement inspired by Friedman. Milton Friedman's classic definition of a universal educational voucher rests on three pillars: the voucher must be available to all students, *regardless of ability or parental income;* students must be eligible for 100 per cent of the public funds that would otherwise be used for private, or public, education; and funds must be 'largely free from government interference.' In other words, the classic definition of an educational voucher is based on universal eligibility, real purchasing power for consumers, and the elimination of barriers to choice of school, whether public or private. States that meet this requirement have, according to the Friedman Foundation, met the 'gold standard' of educational voucher choice.

When presented with lots and lots of options, parents will interview each school, do the background research, and choose the best school for their child's needs. Put differently, school voucher policy acknowledges that the public is not a monolith; that people are diligent in researching their options when the reward is significant; that individual child and family needs differ profoundly; that perceptions of needs differ;

and that one general option, no matter how seemingly ideal, does not satisfy everyone, nor should we ever expect this to be the case.

Educational vouchers exist in both Canada and the United States, provided either by governments or by private donors. In Canada, government-issued vouchers (or 'direct per-student grants') are common in provinces such as Alberta, British Columbia, Manitoba, Quebec, and Saskatchewan. In Ontario, the government does not issue vouchers or tuition tax credits; the only educational voucher available for students in Ontario is a privately funded initiative called Children First: School Choice Trust, which is supported financially by the W. Garfield Weston Foundation. Children First offers tuition assistance grants so that parents who could not otherwise afford it can choose an independent elementary school for their children.

As of the time of writing, in the United States, government-funded scholarships for students are available in six states – Florida, Maine, Ohio, Utah, Vermont, and Wisconsin – as well as the District of Columbia. In a similar vein, tuition tax credits are offered to families in states such as Arizona, Florida, Illinois, Iowa, Minnesota, and Pennsylvania. Tax credits mean that parents receive a dollar-for-dollar reduction in their state income tax liability for every dollar spent on tuition, up to a predetermined limit. Created by Congress in 2004, the Opportunity Scholarship Program (now, as of the time of writing, under threat of White House policy change) is the nation's only federally funded voucher program. It is open to students who live in the Washington school district and whose families have incomes below the federal poverty line – about $40,000 for a family of four. Recipients are chosen by lottery, though preference is given to those attending traditional schools deemed to be in need of improvement under federal law. A federal evaluation in 2009 found that the mostly poor black and Hispanic participants were making major academic gains and narrowing the educational gap with children from wealthy families.

Fiery opposition to educational vouchers exists, sometimes as a result of political ideology. In the United States, voucher opponents – specifically, public school teachers and teachers' unions (notably, the National Education Association, or NEA) – generally oppose school vouchers. In a letter sent to every Democrat in the U.S. House of Representatives and Senate in 2009, the teachers' union wrote: 'Opposition to vouchers is a top priority for NEA.'[156] Opposition to charter schools comes most strongly from public sector unions and from wealthy white liberals concerned about the supposed negative effects on minorities 'left behind' in failing public schools when more fortunate parents move their children away. They fail to see that the ultimate aim of school-based competition through voucher policy is to enable excellent schools for all, rich or poor.

Detractors argue that private schools are too selective and that they discriminate against special needs students and ethnic or racial minorities – despite clear evidence that these groups are precisely the ones that most fervently embrace vouchers. According to critics, providing vouchers for private education is an indirect endorsement of discriminatory educational practices. Some who advocate for the bright-line separation of church and state also oppose government-issued vouchers because many private schools are religiously affiliated. Yet Americans are a highly religious people, so it stands to reason that some would want religion and school integrated.

Our view is that educational vouchers recognize the unique and special needs of students. Attending a school of one's choice is a fundamentally human right, since every child deserves the right to aspire to greatness. After all, education vouchers were introduced because many government-mandated public schools were demonstrably failing millions of American children, particularly those residing in urban black areas. During the 2008–9 school year in America, 61,700 students nationwide received vouchers, up 9 per cent from the previous school year. The growing school choice movement says that educational vouchers will make public schools more accountable because a student could divest his or her student funding to another school if the current school were inadequate. Public schools will be improved by competition. The logic draws on the fundamental insight of the great economist Joseph Schumpeter, who noted that mediocre firms (or here, mediocre failing schools) would be 'creatively destroyed' by competition and that competition would make for continuous improvement in companies (or schools).

Empowering parents generates a competitive education market, which in turn leads to bursts of innovation, niche schools, and overall improvement of all schools. Educational vouchers support the idea of choice for everyone. The universality of the entitlement, as we later describe, addresses the criticism we volley at so many existing obesity management initiatives that, we feel, are perceived as stigmatizing. Vouchers can be enormously varied in their offerings. School vouchers, for example, might pay for transportation to the child's school of choice, for the legumes and lentils at the school of choice, or for a pre-school program at the school of choice.

Outside of education, there has been some policy rhetoric about the power of vouchers, but little implementation in the classic Friedman sense. Some governments have implemented vouchers to reduce indus-trial pollutants. In the European Union, member states receive carbon credits to encourage lower greenhouse gas emissions. In the United States, the 'Cash for Clunkers' program introduced by the Obama White House in 2009 was described as a pollution voucher scheme because the program aimed to promote the purchase of fuel-efficient vehicles. (The purchase of such vehicles evaporated when the program died.) Whether Friedman would have approved of this voucher program is entirely another matter. It put cash in the hands of all consumers, to be sure, but its policy goal was not to give consumers *choice* over where to buy cars (say, as between a government-owned monopoly car store ver-sus a private car store), but simply to stimulate the economy. Friedman would have argued, based on his elemental belief in the power of unfet-tered markets, that a better approach to make this happen would have been broad tax cuts. All things being equal, more cash in the hands of the consumer enables more liberty, more choice.

Healthy Living Vouchers: Focusing on Individual Needs

In health care, vouchers have been used in a very limited sense, and again, not in the classic Friedman way. The only historic reference that we could find to the phrase 'healthy living vouchers' was to a disband-ed 2001 North East Wales 'Carer Information Scheme,' which offered money in a pilot program to eligible adult caregivers who looked after family, partners, or friends in need of help because of long-term ill-ness, disability, or the effects of old age. Though that was in a different context and for a different purpose, the ethos was inspiring to us: give unpaid, generally poor adults (caregivers) money and they will seek out a solution to a highly complex problem (caring for the frail elderly) that works for them.

In the United Kingdom, multiple experiments are under way with a health care voucher scheme that empowers patients with a wide number of conditions such as multiple sclerosis, motor neuron dis-ease, and severe forms of asthma and diabetes to shop around for care, arrange visits when they want, swap one type of treatment for another, or buy their services from the voluntary and private sectors.[157] In other words, the UK's publicly funded National Health Service (NHS) will not place money directly into the hands of patients, but will provide them with more control in terms of deciding how public health care funds are administered. For example, many UK primary health care trusts and health boards operate a voucher scheme for people who are assessed as needing a wheelchair. The program provides for different options with respect to wheelchairs and usually lasts for five years.

Versions of health care vouchers have also been implemented in other countries. In Nicaragua, for example, the state provides sex trade workers with vouchers to obtain free and responsive sexual health services at pre-contracted medical centres. The idea behind the program is to improve access to reproductive health care by giving sex workers a voucher entitling them to free care from any one of between eight and ten private, NGO, and public clinics. The participating clinics are contracted by competitive tender. The women take their vouchers to the clinic of their choice, where they receive the specified services. The clinics then return the vouchers to the agency for reimbursement. The voucher round is repeated every five to six months. Women testing positive for sexually transmitted disease are given an additional voucher, which can be used before the next round. According to independent evaluations, the women now have better access to health care, as well as greater choice. They experience lower rates of perceived stigmatization by clinic staff and feel more empowered than if they were forced into one clinic and had no choice among providers. The incidence of gonorrhea and syphilis has dramatically decreased. On the request of female sex workers, the voucher program has been extended to their partners, pimps, and regular clients – a process that enables the women to negotiate safer sex practices.

So-called vouchers are issued by governments and employers to subsidize child care expenses. The UK currently has what it calls a child care voucher scheme. It is similar to the Canada Child Tax Benefit and the Universal Child Care Benefit administered by Human Resources and Social Development Canada. In Canada, Prime Minister Stephen Harper has started giving parents what some observers have called a voucher in exchange for enrolling their young children in physically active sports at certified organizations. The Child Fitness Tax Credit was launched in 2007 by the Government of Canada with the aim of encouraging children to be more physically active. This non-refundable tax credit is based on eligible fitness expenses paid by parents to register a child in certain physical activity programs. The tax credit allows parents to claim up to C$500 per year in eligible fitness expenses paid for a child under eighteen.

Our Vision of HLVs

Our concept of HLVs, in contrast to subsidies such as the child physical activity benefit, satisfies all three elements of the Friedman model of the classic voucher:

1. Universal eligibility (all persons sixteen and over, thin or obese, are eligible for HLVs).
2. Real purchasing power in the hands of individuals (that is, sufficient funds).
3. The elimination of monopolistic barriers to choice over weight management solutions.

Until now, there has been very limited discussion of true vouchers – or any type of individualized economic incentive – to curb obesity and ensure healthy eating and sustained weight management. But it is instructive to review what's been tried so far that comes close.

In their most basic form, healthy food vouchers have been implemented in different contexts around the world in order to encourage people to take basic nutrients. In sub-Saharan Africa, for instance, the World Food Program launched a food voucher program in February 2009 to combat hunger and the skyrocketing cost of basic food staples in urban areas.[158] The food voucher initiative enables families with young children to purchase food that will boost children's intake of vitamins and minerals. The WFP began the operation for 120,000 people in Ouagadougou in Burkina Faso. A second operation, for 60,000 people, was launched in Bobo-Dioulasso at the end of March 2009. A family typically receives six vouchers a month, each voucher worth about $3 – a significant sum in impoverished countries.

In Syria, the World Food Program has kicked off an electronic food voucher project, using mobile phone technology to help one thousand Iraqi refugee families obtain food.[159] The refugees receive $22 worth of vouchers every two months. Recipients also receive a text message with a code on their mobile phones. The code permits them to go to selected government shops and redeem food items. There are around 130,000 Iraqi refugees in Syria, and they all have mobile phones with no-cost text message functionality.

In the United States, the federal government's Supplemental Nutrition Assistance Program (SNAP) provides low-income and no-income families with what might loosely be referred to as healthy food vouchers. Through nutrition education partners, SNAP helps clients learn to make healthy eating and active lifestyle choices. Similarly, the federal government's Special Supplemental Nutrition Program for Women, Infants, and Children (WIC) provides low-income pregnant women and nursing mothers with vouchers to purchase food items such as eggs, milk, bread, cereal, and formula. Starting in October 2009, the U.S. federal government made nutritional changes to WIC. The food voucher changes allow for the addition of fruits and vegetables and whole grains for the first time for mothers and children aged one to five and allow for baby food fruits and vegetables for infants aged six to twelve months. The rapid growth in obese Americans is why government food stamp programs are placing a greater emphasis on a balanced, nutritional diet. But keep in mind that such programs fail on two elements of the Friedman test: they are not universal (that is, available to all regardless of income), and just as important, they do not expand the range of places from which people can buy their food.

The UK government believes that providing its citizens with incentives will promote healthy living.[160] In January 2008 it introduced a 'voucher-like' strategy to curb the crippling financial costs of obesity. For example, the government encourages employers to implement 'competitions with money, vouchers and other rewards for people who give up junk food in favor of healthy eating and living.' A similar initiative, called 'Pound-for-Pound,' provides obese volunteers in Essex a £1 voucher for every pound they shed.[161] Theoretically, the initiative could produce tangible results, because vouchers are only redeemable for fruits and vegetables at a local grocery store. Though close to the concept of a healthy living voucher, this actually *limits* the places – to one megastore chain, in fact – where people can buy their healthy food. It also limits the ways in which we motivate people to curb their weight loss to just one traditional top-down public health approach: eating more fruits and vegetables.

There are other programs similar in nature to 'healthy living' initiatives, but these schemes differ from the Essex venture. Due to the growing problem of obesity in Ireland, for example, the Gift Voucher Shop – Ireland's largest supplier of gift vouchers – unveiled a holiday voucher scheme called the 'Healthy Alternative Easter Campaign' to combat unhealthy eating habits during holidays such as Easter and Christmas. The Healthy Alternative Easter Campaign encourages citizens to purchase gift vouchers for family vacation resorts that offer children physical activity, instead of providing children with chocolates and sweets on holidays.

The South Korean government provides children with body mass indices near the obesity threshold with a $33 monthly voucher that can be used at a fitness gym.[162] According to the South Korean health minister: 'Kids won't be able to waste the money on eating sweets. We will give them electronic vouchers that can only be used in designated places.' The voucher scheme is believed by many South Koreans to be cost effective because childhood obesity is causing an enormous strain on the country's health care budget. The South Korean and Essex schemes are both noteworthy. In fact, researchers at the University of Pennsylvania have scientifically confirmed the efficacy of small cash incentives on weight loss in limited case studies.[163] But these are not true Friedman-like vouchers since they don't give the people with the cash supplements more options to lose weight than they already have.

Will more substantial HLVs work to combat obesity? We will first describe our approach and then address some of the challenges to it. Vouchers that are universal and that offer people strong and meaningful purchasing power (like Friedman's classical definition of education vouchers) will help reduce stigma because everyone, rich or poor, will be entitled to vouchers (that is, overweight people will not be targeted). This in turn will provide better and more tangible returns for our health care dollars. Another approach is to 'means test' participants, but this would violate the Friedman principle and potentially exacerbate stigma. (As we argue later, we welcome jurisdictions to adjust the HLV policy as they see fit, and means testing is one such adaptation whose impact is worth exploring.) Since our model treats the voucher as taxable income, the early adopters may more likely be the poor in lower tax brackets. Imagine what could be done if a pilot study gave participants $5,000 per year – not an inconceivable sum when we consider the size of health care budgets in industrialized countries. The amount would be used during the year, with the patient committing in writing, with his or her primary care provider, to follow through on an individualized weight management plan. This policy would liberate patients and their providers to choose an option that works; it would also hold both parties accountable for results in a non-stigmatizing and non-threatening way. Drawing on the insights of economist Cecil Pigou, we believe that certain economic activities, such as the purchase of goods and services to sustain a healthy lifestyle, have tremendous social value. The benefits in productivity, human health, prevention, and stigma reduction far outweigh the immediate capital investment.

Under an HLV system, people would enjoy the freedom to shop around – working together with their primary care provider – and to choose the best means, for them, by which they could lose or stabilize weight. Obesity policy, we feel, doesn't need to constrain liberty through taxation or regulation; indeed, it can enhance it. By empowering everyone to decide how best to spend a specified sum of healthy living dollars to maintain a healthy lifestyle, the state would be transforming obesity policy into one that is proactive, that focuses on long-term health, that partners with industry, and that is inclusive – even fun – in contrast to current policy, which is reactionary, stigmatizing, and often antagonistic toward industry. Of the pot-pourri of available options tailored to the individual, many can be pleasurable – ideally, just as pleasurable as consuming food itself.

An HLV makes possible a wide net of weight loss and weight management choices, recognizing that everyone is an individual and requires help with obesity ('N of 1') either now or in the future; pretty much everyone is today, or tomorrow, at risk of tipping the scales too far in the wrong direction. As such, it falls on the individual, working with his or her primary care provider, to determine whether the HLV should be used for a gym membership, sleep therapy, nutrition lessons, Bikram yoga (which might sweat out 750 calories per session), ballet, gardening, golf or cooking lessons, spas, physiotherapy, massage, chiropody, hip hop dancing, peer-to-peer counselling, the purchase of Wii sports games and consoles, iPods equipped with pedometers, or technical applications for glucose monitoring. The list does not end there. The *participatory and accountable journey* to a weight loss option is what matters.

Central to the joint decision over which weight loss option to try would be an ongoing, reflective joint investigation, involving both the patient and the primary care provider, into what might motivate the patient to trim down. For example, for some elderly people, personal health benefits may matter less than decreasing the financial and emotional burden of their ill health on the next generation (that is, their sons or daughters). They may be best motivated to lose weight within the framework of 'generativity,' a term coined by the psychoanalyst Erik Erikson in 1950 to denote 'a concern for establishing and guiding the next generation.'

Ideally, people will choose something they enjoy – this is of great importance if they're going to maintain it – and something they and their care provider believe will work for them based on a detailed examination of available options. To take but one example, more than 50 million Wii consoles were sold between 2006 and 2009. Researchers have found that people expend more energy playing some Wii sports games, notably Wii Fit and Wii Boxing, than taking a brisk walk. People who buy Wii consoles are self-selected; they're the people who enjoy video games.

Stripping away society's preconceived notions of what constitutes 'exercise' – and what motivates different people to exercise and shed weight – will be essential to the success of any HLV policy. If the choice doesn't work for the patient, the patient and his or her primary care provider can switch course. Of course, not every option that someone might want will be made available; too much weight loss quackery exists. Options need to be vetted by a self-regulatory certification process, which we will address below.

Doctors or other primary care providers would be available to help patients choose from a wide array of certified anti-obesity programs. To ensure independence, certification could be done by a legislated, self-regulating group led by a board or college representing the perspectives of all regulated health professions in any given province or state – dentists, physicians, nurses, midwives, traditional Chinese medical doctors (if the latter are regulated in the jurisdiction), and so forth. The multiple, essential in-person and online discussions between patient and provider on weight management topics and options would be reimbursed by the state or insurer. In a publicly funded health care model, reimbursement to the primary care provider could come through new, specialized billing codes for sustained obesity management – that is, 'healthy living counselling.' The government could mandate minimum reimbursement in the case of a private insurance company, but the insurer or provider network would negotiate a fair rate for the provider–patient discussion as a way to encourage take-up and increased illness prevention and patient self-management.

The potential of HLVs to work seamlessly within private insurance or publicly funded health care models is important. HLVs, because they must be spent every year, would be very different from health savings accounts, or HSAs, which are tax-favoured medical savings accounts available to taxpayers in the United States who are enrolled in a high-deductible health plan. Funds contributed to HSAs are not subject to federal income tax at the time of deposit and can accumulate tax-free over time. Proponents of HSAs, variants of which have been tried in

Singapore and South Africa and the United States, believe that they are an important reform that will help reduce the growth of health care costs and increase the efficiency of the health care system. HSAs, it is argued, encourage saving for future health care expenses, allowing the patient to receive needed care without an insurance gatekeeper to determine which benefits are allowed; in that way, HSAs make consumers more responsible for their own health care choices. Opponents of HSAs say they worsen the health system's problems because healthy people will leave insurance plans while sick people will avoid HSAs. There is also debate about consumer satisfaction with HSAs.

For the purposes of preventing obesity, HSAs are potentially problematic because they may encourage people to delay prevention. This is one reason why groups like the American Public Health Association and Consumers Union oppose them. This may be a concern in the matter of obesity, since the deadliest effects of increased obesity, such as heart attack and stroke and cancer, do not surface for many years. The pharmacotherapy of obesity through drugs like Lipitor exaggerates this delay. That said, we do not want to impugn HSAs or their opposite – nationally insured systems like Canada's – both of which have benefits and drawbacks from the perspective of equity, cost, administrative efficiency, and medical innovation. Our concern here is to develop an HLV model that is able to combat obesity within *any* existing funding model. One benefit, therefore, of allowing different jurisdictions to adjust and pilot HLVs is to enable a kind of natural experiment that may indicate whether a particular funding formula improves outcomes.

HSAs assign full responsibility to the consumer; HLVs meet the consumer halfway, respecting him as an individual with specific weight loss challenges while at the same time compelling him to make weight management decisions in conjunction with his health care provider under the rules of a regulatory regime sanctioned by government legislative oversight and by a regulatory college. HLVs do not favour any particular government funding model, be it fully public (national health insurance for all services, as in Cuba), semi-private hybrid model (as in Sweden or Germany), or fully private, as under the HSA model envisioned in the Medicare Prescription Drug, Improvement, and Modernization Act, which was signed into law by President George W. Bush in December 2003.

One benefit of an HLV scheme is that it would increase competition among a wide assortment of healthy living service providers, from specialized gyms to grocery chains to technology companies to home retrofitting businesses. By opening our eyes to the fact that a massive swath of the general service sector has a direct impact on our health choices and on our weight, this policy will abruptly arouse brisk competition among such service providers to attract valuable voucher dollars. The ensuing competition and innovation in the private sector could more than make up for any early HLV dollars expended by the state. This would nurture what we referred to earlier as 'creative destruction,' Joseph Schumpeter's concept that the more innovative, more client-friendly industries will necessarily win out in the new marketplace over the long term.

Anticipating Objections to HLVs

1. *Where Does the Money Come From?*

HLVs are an untried policy idea – a hypothesis based on a number of assumptions and observations described in this book. So we recommend that jurisdictions around the world try a pilot project first, prior to full-scale launch. A pilot would need to pre-certify a wide range of weight loss options but would inevitably offer far fewer choices than full-scale HLV implementation. In making the jump from consideration of HLVs to commitment to the HLV model, a number of policy considerations would need to be more fully addressed. We consider what we believe may be the leading objections here, looking at the policy challenges and the associated opportunities.

For any voucher for healthy living to be meaningful, it will have to be substantial in sum and ongoing, recognizing the immense costs of obesity in terms of human health, notably chronic illness. Every dollar spent in the form of a voucher, if wisely spent to prevent the burden of obesity, would add enormous wealth to government budgets and save private and public insurers money in the long run. We propose that at least 10 per cent of the health budget in developed countries – this being just a portion of the total direct and indirect monies spent on health – be reallocated to cash vouchers redeemable to anyone who is properly committed to healthy living, who, working intimately with a primary care provider, will be entitled to spend the money for weight loss or weight management.

Ten per cent of the health care budget sounds like a lot of money. Yet in industrialized countries, about 10 per cent (and rising) annually of health care budgets get swallowed up by obesity-related health problems. Obesity-related costs may even be as high as 20 per cent, as noted in chapter 1. Consider that Canada's health care expenditures exceed $180 billion and that they are surging at a rate of 5.5 per cent per year. In the United Kingdom, health care accounted for 8.4 per cent of GDP in 2007. The UK's GDP in 2007 was estimated to be $2.21 trillion, and health care expenditures in 2007 came in at $263 billion.

Looking more closely at the U.S. data, we see that in 2009, direct health care costs amounted to at least $2.3 trillion. Health care represents one-seventh of the entire U.S. economy. About 70 per cent of that relates to individuals' choices and behaviours. Beyond the $2.3+ trillion, several hundreds of billions get spent on public health – which includes everything from the wasteful public education campaigns discussed throughout this book, to critical vaccination and water fluoridation. Roughly 5 per cent of the U.S. health budget is spent on health promotion. Since data on health care expenditures are fuzzy, depending on what we mean by 'health care' – for example, does this include employer benefit costs, like gym memberships? – let's round up the total U.S. health budget to roughly $3 trillion. That means that 10 per cent of the total health budget gets us to $300 billion, which is a considerable sum of money. With $300 billion annually, the U.S. government could offer roughly $1,900 per year per person over the age of fifteen for HLVs (there were roughly 155 million Americans over fifteen as of 2010). For a family of four, this would be $7,600 – initially to begin as a pilot project to evaluate its impact. For many families and individuals, this offset would reduce their health costs considerably. (If the amount were graduated according to family income – an option we discuss later – this subsidy could rise substantially for the poorest families.)

Without revisiting the staggering cost burdens associated with obesity, it would be remiss to forget some basic facts about why Western industrialized health care systems are hitting the wall financially. Thanks in large part to extraordinarily expensive but life-saving and life-altering medical technologies concentrated at the end of life, health care is draining the public purse. By any generally accepted accounting principle, industrialized health care systems are bankrupt. Many jurisdictions are facing the reality of insufficient care providers – nurses, diabetes specialists, cardiologists, gerontologists, psychologists, oncologists, psychiatrists, general practitioners, surgeons, palliative care physicians – to take care of the current crop of frail elderly citizens, much less to provide for generations of chronically ill people to come.

The policy debate, therefore, is less about the extraordinary cost savings that would ensue from taking better care of our bodies – to which the vast consensus of clinicians, economists, policy makers, and even politicians pay lip service – than about moving from rhetoric to reality. How are we to make what Richard Thaler and Cass Sunstein call 'the nudge' work when it comes to obesity?[164] If HLVs are the answer to ensuring the 'nudge,' then there have to be sufficient funds to bring it about. We suggested earlier that U.S. policy makers peg $1,900 per year for every person above the age of consent (generally stipulated at age sixteen in the context of health care, though this varies and is often not legislated but rather governed by the common law). One legitimate concern is that this may be too low a sum. As we have argued, the payments must be substantial in order to motivate individuals and their primary care providers, and they must be large enough to create a vibrant marketplace where companies can compete for certification and gain access to consumers' voucher dollars. We will therefore consider a way to get to more substantial amounts of funding, but first we must deal with the issue of quackery.

2. *How Do We Prevent Quack Treatments?*

The source of voucher money should be the state. Though our public health policy solution embraces the power of markets to offer alternative weight loss solutions, it relies on self-regulatory bodies to ensure proper certifications. The state must play a crucial role in setting the rules, standards, and governance requirements – through umbrella legislation supported by the public – to which self-regulatory bodies (such as a state's regulatory College of Nurses) must adhere. This will limit representation in the certification group to all pre-existing regulated health care professions in the jurisdiction, which will in turn limit fringe treatments that have absolutely no perceived evidence base (for example, tanning salons for weight loss). It will also balance the interests of the represented clinician provider groups – for instance, by preventing physicians from crowding out the opinions of naturopaths (assuming that naturopaths are already regulated by the state). Should, over time, new health care professions be regulated in any jurisdiction, such as midwives (whose current legal status varies greatly among jurisdictions), a representative from this profession would be entitled to sit, with equal influence, on the certification council.

This approach means that the actual certification threshold of acceptability of services would inevitably vary from country to country, state to state, and province to province. Yet the federal government could stipulate standards through the enabling legislation – by, for example, stipulating the governance and decision rules by which certification decisions should be made and reconsidered (say, on a biannual basis). Because jurisdictions will enjoy flexibility in implementation, HLVs would be more politically saleable. The best precedent for this in the health care sector is regulated medical and nursing and dental colleges, which, throughout much of the industrialized world – notably in Canada and the UK – operate autonomously but under basic guidelines or principles that are legislated.

Within the ambit of such state regulation, ours is hardly a radical, libertarian policy idea, though it is laissez-faire in structure. At the same time, we believe it important that the state combat obesity without becoming a 'nanny state,' since, as we have argued, public health officials' powers of 'persuasion' are weak to non-existent. The state must be on the hook financially because taxpayers are already too burdened and are already paying for their neighbours' weight problems. Your neighbour's weight already affects how much you pay in state or provincial taxes for any government service, notably public school education from junior kindergarten through to public university. The great untold story in the rise of health care costs globally is the rapid clip with which health costs are now eating into our ability to pay for good teachers to educate our children from kindergarten through to university. Obesity today is ripping into society's basic education rights, which, as we have suggested, are essential to liberty.

3. *How Do We Get Enough Funds to Sustain HLVs?*

To find more monies for HLVs, the ideal system would take a portion of the *entire government budget*, not just a portion of the health care budget. Such an approach is logically consistent with the overall science of obesity, which, while unsettled, recognizes that obesity is 'multipronged.' Instead of drawing away 10 per cent of the health care budget, therefore, or a higher percentage of the public health portion of the health budget, the better solution to pay for HLVs may be to hive away 2 to 4 per cent of the entire government budget to pay for them, in particular, for the pilot round. This should satisfy many researchers and policy makers, who acknowledge, correctly, that sectors as diverse as education, social services, energy, and the environment all play a role in fighting obesity. To single out the health department or ministry for funding HLVs would thus be narrow minded. Applying HLV monies from the global government budget would also circumvent the administrative challenges of asking one ministry or department to administer the HLV fund.

If the HLV money is a 2 to 4 per cent slice off the entire government budget, then funds could be allocated through a simple provincial or state tax cut; or through a direct cash payment to taxpayers. It should fall on the state or province to decide for itself the most efficient manner in which to pilot, pay for, and administer HLVs. Like the Congressional Opportunity Scholarship Program, HLVs could be implemented by states in such a way that individuals over a certain age, or parents, receive a dollar-for-dollar reduction in their state tax for every dollar spent on certified healthy living services, up to a predetermined limit. Another approach might be to experiment with success-contingent vouchers, which compel recipients after, say, five years to give back their voucher dollars with accumulated interest if they fail to succeed in compliance (for example, to meet with their primary care provider physically or by virtual means four times annually). Means testing for lower-income candidates only would open up more funds for those eligible but would also violate the Friedman principle of universal eligibility; encounter sustained stigma; and fail to recognize that all people (except the megarich) are at considerable risk for obesity (even if the poor may be more so). Nonetheless, as mentioned, we welcome states to experiment with means testing in the context of HLVs, especially if this is a pilot policy in staged implementation. Alternatively, all people sixteen and over might be eligible, with higher levels of HLV funding offered to the poorest members of society.

To compel people to pay back the government entirely for failing to reduce weight would be too punitive and would, we feel, severely limit uptake of HLVs. Furthermore, this approach might be too similar to merit-based aid for college and university applicants, with all the shortcomings of such programs – it would inevitably motivate the wealthier, more driven, more educated classes. We recognize that merit-based aid in the education field may have compelling counter-arguments (in contrast, for example, to need-based aid for college and university students, which does little to improve incentives for academic performance). In the case of HLVs, however, it is critical to avoid the self-selection of participants, since we want these HLVs to help people of all incomes, especially considering that low-income individuals are relatively more at risk for obesity. The potential benefits of HLVs must be spread as widely as possible.

4. *How Do We Enable Flexibility in HLV Programs?*

As noted earlier in the context of means testing, it is possible for jurisdictions to enjoy the flexibility of offering people the choice of payback schedules, such that people receive more voucher dollars if they take the risk of failure to drop weight; or if they risk the failure to manage their weight according to preset goals agreed upon with their primary care provider. If his clients do well, the primary care provider could win out, in the form of a bonus of continuing medical education credits or a cash subsidy or some type of public or professional recognition. Inspiration for this idea comes from a twist on the notion of income-contingent loans for certain U.S. college students, who must give back loans from a portion of future earnings. Under our twist, voucher recipients would not need to give back their dollars if they complied in showing sustained interaction and communication with their primary care provider; and they could keep their 'winnings' if, according to the care providers, they surpassed mutually agreed upon goals.

Admittedly, there are other challenges to our proposed HLV scheme that need to be explored. First, government bureaucrats and health care practitioners might object because a portion of health care funds would inevitably move to the less regulated private sector. Some might object to this on grounds of patient safety; others on grounds of ideology or ethics. This, therefore, would demand a strong legislated regulatory body for certification, as discussed earlier. If everyone chose to apply their vouchers for certified gym memberships, what would happen to the income of diabetes nurses or reimbursement for bariatric obesity surgeons? We feel that the labour market would dynamically sort this problem out. As an added benefit, the true value of a private diabetes nurse, or a post-operative community-based coach for the obese, would be more demonstrable after HLVs. This is Schumpeterian 'creative destruction' at work. Consumers would signal through market demand the deserved wage levels of all weight-management health providers, tools, and devices.

Another issue to address head-on is implementation: How will the HLV policy be implemented from province to province or from state to state (or, in the UK, from trust to trust), considering that in federated countries such as Canada and the United States, health care is the responsibility of provinces and states? Should every jurisdiction offer the same program, or could they differ? One answer is that the federal government could set standards (for example, the broad categories of service provider organizations to be qualified as weight loss organizations), but it would be for each province, trust, or state to administer its own program through the legislated, self-regulatory authority referred to earlier, and to set minimums at which provider–patient weight management discussions would be reimbursed.

5. *How Do We Prevent Abuses?*

There is another potential challenge to HLVs: How will the state ensure that citizens are using the vouchers appropriately and not fraudulently? In other words, you can subsidize someone's gym membership, but you cannot mandate that same individual to attend the gym for the purpose of exercise rather than meeting up with friends, drinking at the juice bar, and socializing. Providing vouchers would definitely empower citizens. But empowerment can only go so far; citizens must also be held *accountable*, otherwise empowerment will mean little. Accountability comes in at the point of care – that is, at the relationship between the primary care provider and the patient. A certificate of attendance should be required yearly. To qualify for ongoing voucher money, patients should need to input bimonthly (or more frequent) online status updates about their weight management activities. The state can – and should – demand annual physical examinations with a primary care provider, and the patient needs to consent and commit to follow through on the weight management program, and mutually set goals, to which she and her provider commit.

6. *How Do We Ensure a Patient's Commitment?*

At the next annual physical, or at an interim appointment held online, a participatory discussion can take place about the program's effectiveness. Utilizing personal health records shared between a doctor and a patient (in the form of templates such as Microsoft's Healthvault or Google Health), it is easy for the parties to make these evaluations on an ongoing basis online. Each evaluation and discussion, be it online (perhaps through Skype) or via in-person consults, must be reimbursable to the primary care provider; and it must be the dual responsibility of the patient and the doctor to switch plans if the first-choice healthy living option is not showing signs of promise. If it's not working and there's no switch, the money stops. HLVs thereby combat obesity by treating people like rational, unique adults while recognizing that people aren't always rational when it comes to eating and exercising.

A lesson from behavioural economists studying the actions of stroke victims is instructive here. After a stroke, doctors usually prescribe a blood thinner to help reduce the chance of recurrence from 24 per cent to 4 per cent. Even though taking this drug significantly reduces the possibility of further brain damage, many patients don't take their medicine. In one test group study, twenty patients had an electronic pillbox in their homes that recorded whether they were compliant. If they had not taken their pills correctly, they were disqualified from entering a daily lottery. All participants had a one in five chance of winning a $10 prize in the lottery, and a one in one hundred chance of winning a $100 prize. Winners who had not taken their medication were informed that because they had not complied with the drug regimen, they would receive nothing. Non-compliance dropped from 22 per cent to under 2 per cent for the entire three months of the study.

With state-funded HLVs, it is possible to make the potential rewards for compliance, as well as the consequences for non-compliance, simpler to administer. A patient who failed to participate in the regular HLV re-evaluation process with his primary care provider would enjoy no further eligibility. If we can motivate potential stroke victims with an expected value of just $3 for the lottery described above (based on the probability of winning either of the two lotteries), then surely we can motivate people to keep their commitment to HLVs if there is far more money on the line.

7. What about Low-Income Neighbourhoods?

An additional challenge for HLVs is lack of access to appropriate resources in poor neighbourhoods. An HLV might well be of less utility in a neighbourhood with few grocery stores selling fruit and vegetables, no dance studio, no gym, and no private swimming facilities. For instance, in many inner-city neighbourhoods across Canada and the United States, fresh fruits and vegetables are not readily available in poor areas. How will vouchers benefit people who reside in inner cities, where there are very few healthy food alternatives or activity centres?

Part of the answer may lie in thinking creatively about how people spend and apportion their vouchers. For example, the voucher could be applied to subway or cab fare if access to the metro enables poor people to physically reach a gym (and this evaluation could be made in conjunction with the care provider). Or, people in the inner city might pool their cash vouchers – after all, it's their money to do with as they wish, provided that their primary care provider approves – to build or subsidize a new community hockey rink, bowling alley, basketball court, or recreation centre. Furthermore, when a government sees an HLV-funded project – such as a recreation centre – gaining support in a poor neighbourhood, it can institute a policy to match the funds. This approach can amount to a citizen-driven 'market test' for the projected value of planned government-funded community projects meant to inspire people to be physically active. This is the very opposite of a top-down policy approach: it is creative, 'bottom-up' policy.

Surveying the World: Tax and Shame versus HLVs

To assess public attitudes on the proper role of the state in combating obesity, we surveyed over 53,000 people around the world using an online survey tool. Ours was the first international survey in history that compared people's preferences for one government obesity policy versus another.

We wanted to understand whether people were more favourable to state tactics that gave people financial incentives to lose weight, or to state tactics that prodded them to lose weight. We questioned people's attitudes toward five types of policy, asking them to select one as best:

1. Limit the state's role to education: tell citizens to 'eat right and exercise' by advertising campaigns.
2. Demand that the state impose heavier taxes on obese people.
3. Demand that the state impose heavier taxes on fast food / junk food / caloric food.
4. Provide HLVs tailored to individual weight management needs.
5. No policy at all.

In the hundred-plus countries we surveyed, people were significantly more interested in options 1, 2, and 3 than in option 4. Surveying a random sample of 53,706 English-speaking people in the U.S., Canada, the UK, and around the world between 6 December 2009 and 24 January 2010, we found that 17 per cent preferred HLVs to all the other options. We then zeroed in on six countries of interest, though we looked at more than one hundred countries. These countries of interest were the UK (the most obese European country), China (the most populous),

Turkey (where obesity is on a rapid climb), India (with the highest obesity-related diabetes rate in the world), and the U.S. and Canada (countries grappling with severe rates of obesity). More than half our global sample consisted of people eighteen and older from these countries. It was possible to vote only once in the survey.

We chose to include in our six countries of interest people from India and China, the two most populous countries in the world, both with fast-rising rates of obesity. We aimed for a balance of countries with individualistic cultures – Canada, the UK, and the U.S. – and countries that were more communitarian (China, India, and Turkey). In Turkey, the country's weight problems have skyrocketed as the country has migrated from a highly agrarian society to an industrialized one. In each of these six countries there is official state recognition of the costs to society and to human health arising from the obesity epidemic.

We surveyed a random sample of 30,746 people in these six countries of interest. In the U.S., Canada, and (especially) the UK, taxing the obese for their gluttony was by far the preferred policy option. Among our six countries of interest, this option was most popular in Britain, where 33 per cent of people favoured it. This policy option was significantly less popular among English-speaking respondents in India, where obesity is also an epidemic.

By contrast, mass marketing campaigns ('eat your fruits and vegetables!') were more popular in the industrializing countries – Turkey (24 per cent), China (24 per cent), and India (32 per cent). This makes intuitive sense: these countries have had only limited experimentation with these marketing tools and techniques despite having recognized the pervasiveness of obesity. These nations' citizens are therefore less sensitive to the weaknesses of generic messaging campaigns. Since they are more politically saleable policy options, it makes sense that people in these countries endorsed them.

About 16 per cent of English-speaking survey respondents in the six countries said 'none of the above.' HLVs were a popular policy option among Turkish (20 per cent) and Chinese (23 per cent) respondents. That HLVs registered consistently above 13 per cent in popularity was illuminating. We did not expect this. There is clearly an appetite for this policy option, despite its novelty and its immediate negative effect on the public purse.

In short, our global survey bucketed four types of public policy tools for the state: a carrot (HLVs); a stick (taxing fast food); a bludgeon (taxing the fat); or a bully pulpit (social marketing). We asked this question during the economic downturn of 2009–10, and as such, the findings in support of HLVs may be conservative, since the survey questioned people about policies whose impact would mean spending scarce public funds.

It did not surprise us that anti–fast-food policies and educational marketing initiatives – the status quo – received high levels of support. And the most heavily supported policy was also the most stigmatizing: imposing heavier taxes on fat people. *The UK, the fattest country in Europe, was the most inclined to favour taxing the obese more!* Twenty-eight per cent of Americans picked this, as did 25 per cent of Canadians. There was no statistically significant regional variation within any country. So this meant that places where people were fit (like British Columbia or Colorado) were just as likely to choose the policy stick or the bludgeon as were people in portlier jurisdictions (like Mississippi or Tennessee).

As we have argued, there is a deeply ingrained cultural inclination across North America and the Western world toward punishing the obese via word or wallet, and taxation is one prominent example of this. People generally fail to recognize that this policy would do little except drive already depressed, overweight people away from medical help and thereby exacerbate the problem. Furthermore, the obese already may be paying extra medical costs. Overweight workers are already being paid less than similarly qualified workers, according to research by Jay Bhattacharya and Kate Bundorf of Stanford.[165] The size of the wage differential is similar to the size of the differential between their medical costs and those of the non-obese.

Finally, the very notion of taxing particular products in order to alter behaviour is bad tax policy and bad social engineering. Such targeted tax increases – an obesity plastic surgery tax, a fast foods and chocolate and soda pop tax, a video games tax, all of which have been considered in America and the UK – do little to reduce obesity rates, but they do give government more control over our lives. A 'fat tax' is just not the answer. Penalizing people for their excess weight will not reduce waistlines. The Danish government has come down punishingly hard in the past year: a 25 per cent tax increase on ice cream, chocolate, sweets, and soft drinks. The CDC director Thomas Frieden and many within the public health bureaucracy elite often cite the smoking precedent to support this sin tax idea,[166] but if we followed that example, we'd be starting along a path that leads to measuring waistlines (as in Japan), electronic monitoring of people's movements (as we do with some pris-

Figure 1: Global preferences for different roles for the state in obesity policy

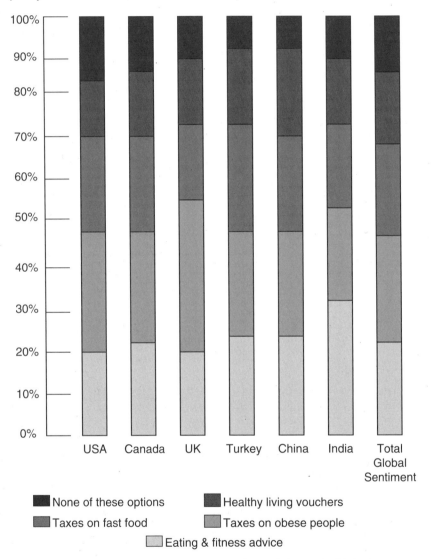

N = 53,706 (Global), N = 12,857 (US), N = 7,355 (Canada), N = 3,288 (Turkey), N = 2,005 (UK), N = 2,777 (China), N = 2,464 (India). Source: Health Strategy Innovation Cell / RIWI Corporation, December 2009–January 2010.

oners), and banning the obese from restaurants (as was seriously considered in Mississippi).

Figure 1 shows the relative popularity of each policy option as expressed by the random sample surveyed. Around the world, imposing taxes on fat people – a policy of shame – generally came out on top. The shaming options in Figure 1 include taxing the obese and barking at people to lose weight.

It is to be expected that a new policy such as HLVs would take time to gain traction in public opinion. There is a precedent, and again, it is school vouchers and charter schools. Consider charter schools. As of late 2009, there were five thousand charters operating in thirty-nine states and the District of Columbia. More than 1.5 million American students attended charters, an 11 per cent increase from 2008. Though that is only 3 per cent of all U.S. public school students, the number has more than quadrupled since 2000. More important, supply is not meeting demand. In June 2009, 365,000 American students were on waiting lists for charter schools.

Historically, it has taken time for the public to embrace school vouchers, given entrenched opposition from the school unions. And there is a long way to go to bring the public fully on board, even though in some jurisdictions, such as Alberta, support for school choice runs high. And despite rising support for school vouchers among poor, visible minorities most in need of school choice, other groups have been more reticent. In the earliest U.S. referenda on the topic of school choice during the 1960s and 1970s, opposition was consistently high in rural areas, in small towns, and on college campuses.[167] Among the urban poor, however, there was immediate interest and early enthusiasm. We would expect to see the same trend with HLVs.

Why do HLVs not immediately capture the public's overwhelming favour? There are several reasons why the idea of HLVs may not immediately resonate with some. First, as we have noted, many wrongly believe that obesity is strictly a matter of personal failure and lack of willpower. As a result, these very same individuals – the majority of whom, statistically, are overweight themselves though they may not admit it – would instead favour draconian health policies such as a fat tax or humiliation. Yet as we know, obesity is a complex social issue – one that is related, among other things, to the ready availability of unhealthy foods as well as to genetics. Second, perhaps people simply object to the notion of using scarce public funds to aid the obese. To many people, HLVs may look a lot like government handouts. Third, health care practitioners and their guild associations may object to an HLV scheme because it would divest public health care funds into the private sector and toward 'competitor' professionals – that is, toward non-regulated health professionals (such as fitness instructors) or (worse!) to private company vendors (such as IBM or Apple or Research In Motion, whose technologies support health self-monitoring tools). Self-interested financially, health care practitioners may oppose HLVs for fear of job insecurity.

Healthy Living Vouchers: Busting Up Vested Interests

In the field of education, vouchers delegate to parents the decision making about schools for their children, wresting it from bureaucrats and unions. That makes some people uncomfortable. And HLVs may make some people uncomfortable as well.

Educational vouchers undermine conventional policy wisdom in the sense that public education has historically been considered the right- ful domain of governments and bureaucrats. In other words, the gener- al public has seen the state as the saviour of universal public education. There was, and still is, the fear that a freer market could undermine the universality of public education, turning it into a privilege acces- sible only to the children of wealthy elites. This makes perfect sense in the minds of many educators, as education was accessible only to the wealthy before it emerged as a universal human right in Western society.

Not so long ago, health was also a privilege. Only the wealthy could afford health care. But it has emerged as a universal legal right in most industrialized countries, as it should be. Despite challenges in access to care for the poor, as a matter of law in the industrialized world, no one showing up sick at a hospital emergency room for whatever reason – including an episode of obesity-related illness, such as an attack of asthma or a diabetic crisis – will ever be turned away. To turn someone away in such circumstances would be to commit legal negligence. Set- ting aside the thorny and politically sensitive issue of a right to publicly funded health insurance, the legal right to basic health is universal in Western nations; but, once sick with obesity-related illness, one can- not always choose one's own treatment path. Some treatments may be unaffordable. When it comes to the prevention of disease caused by obesity, there should be universality, and morally, there should be a right to choose from among a wide number of funded options to get you to good health. That ounce of prevention can take many equally valid forms. Universal HLVs can make that morally correct dream possible.

Preventive, participatory, and accountable health strategies should be selected by individuals from a host of choices. Yes, some may choose unwisely if the field is left completely open. That is where scientific validation and provider hand holding come in. Available options need to have a plausible evidence base as determined by the self-regulatory accrediting body described earlier. As the scientific base for obesity prevention tools and treatments accumulates, only those choices that show sustained evidence of effectiveness among some people will be honoured by the accrediting authority. However, this 'evidence' is, as we have shown, in constant flux and hotly debated. It is also deeply individual. In other words, methods may work for some and not for others. The marketplace – with consumers and primary care providers working together to organically define market demand – will over time define which classes of interventions are the most effective for the greatest numbers of people. What matters is that dubious and dangerous treatments will be cast aside.

Can the system be abused? Yes, initially. Some physicians, sympathizing with their welfare recipient patients, have been known to sign paperwork that allows their patients to collect extra money for ailments such as diabetes, food allergies, and gout without confirming that they actually have those conditions. For example, in Toronto, the city's welfare office in 2009 rejected 'special dietary allowance' requests from Dr Roland Wong, who allegedly signed an unknown number of the forms dating back to 2004, when he obliged a request from the Ontario Coalition Against Poverty, an advocacy group, to vouch for everyone who requested the allowance.[168] Ontario's Special Diet Allowance, which helps very poor people on welfare manage medical conditions, provides up to $250 per month for people suffering from more than forty medical conditions. A 2010 provincial auditor's report said there is evidence that allowance is being abused. So it is to be anticipated that people may try, theoretically, to find ways of buying prescribed illicit substances (and selling them) using their HLVs. Clearly, certification processes will be hotly debated. Will quack treatments be certified? Perhaps, initially, but not for long once trial lawyers start suing abusive weight management organizations, just as they routinely sue disreputable, unhygienic nursing homes in class action, contingency-fee lawsuits.

Free choice market economies can and should champion choice in illness prevention. Enterprises entered into freely are the most likely to succeed. Vouchers promote competition among providers and participatory medicine, just as school vouchers promote the rise of best-in-class schools and engaged parents. They are based on sound economic principles and can honour evolving scientific, evidential, and clinical expertise. A voucher system for healthy living recognizes that we are all free moral agents; that we all have individual obesity challenges; that the causes of obesity are complex and many; that obesity is a lifelong challenge; and that we can take time and want the time to experiment with what works best for us, for our families, and for those whom we love.

What we have learned in this book is that mass market campaigns to encourage people to hew to 'healthy weights' just aren't 'sticking,' as advertising mavens would say. People who work in state public health positions genuinely want to do good work; they have invariably given up higher-paying positions in the for-profit sector for the opportunity to do good work. But they seem to be preoccupied with what should work at a *system level* rather than what *does* work in fighting obesity at an individual level. And in targeting the policy forest, they neglect the trees.

Measuring Individual Success

HLV commitments may work best if there is a downside to failing and an upside to succeeding. There are some examples to consider when introducing accountability for results. For instance, StickK.com is a hugely popular website that motivates people to make changes in their lives by gambling on their reputation. If they fail to achieve self-advertised goals, they're out pocket for the money and their significant others know it. In February 2009, the site had more than twenty-three thousand users, the highest percentage of whom (42 per cent) had made commitment contracts to lose weight. The Commitment Contract concept is based on two principles:

1. People don't always do what they set out to do.
2. Incentives work if tailored to individual desires.

The website takes credit card information up front and charges the user's card weekly if he fails (by self-report) to meet his self-declared personal goal. StickK.com users set up whatever goals they like and have the option of putting as much money at stake as they want. They usually designate a 'referee' (a friend, coworker, or spouse), who receives regular progress e-mails.

Forfeited money from unfulfilled promises goes to a charity or, depending on the user's preference, an 'anti-charity' – one that the user doesn't support. For example, a person who is against abortion can designate the NARAL Pro-Choice America Foundation as the recipient if he fails to meet his personal goal. About 85 to 90 per cent of users fulfil their contracts, but that, of course, is by self-report. There's not much shame involved because it is private, and if they fail, the money goes (secretly) to a good cause (or a 'bad' cause, as the case may be). Such experiments are exciting because they allow individuals to regulate privately the way they want to behave. In the Philippines, this approach has been a success with smokers who wanted to quit: after depositing money into a zero-interest account, they got their money back six months later if they passed a test showing they had stayed nicotine-free for six months. If they failed, a charity got the cash.[169]

It is now possible to track individual success like never before. New York City has a way of monitoring all its citizens diagnosed with diabetes. Medical laboratories in New York forward the results of thousands of blood sugar tests to the city Health Department, which analyses the data and identifies those whose diabetes is out of control. Patients then receive prods, letters, or phone calls from their doctors, reminding them to take medication, come in for a check-up, change their diet, or exercise more. And this kind of tracking and prodding can be individualized using an HLV model where a primary care provider and patient connect virtually in ways they choose and that fit comfortably into their life routines. For those who fail to honour their pledge to monitor and report their progress, future HLV dollars can be cut off. In this way, technology (here, no-cost cellphone text messaging) emerges as a kind of wireless health monitoring, delivering personalized health information, evaluating the success of jointly selected interventions, and keeping channels of communication open between people at home or at work and their health care providers.

Everyone Has a Personal Story of Weight Loss

Tired of the conflicting reports coming out of the peer-reviewed obesity research and the mainstream media, colleagues at the Health Strategy Innovation Cell (at the University of Toronto's Massey College) used

Web 'listening' technology to determine what people were saying online about their personal solutions to weight loss and weight management. People write about these stories on blogs and social networks devoted to talking about personal challenges. There are millions of these personal narratives on the Web. Innovation Cell research has found that people write on blogs about highly stigmatized conditions – notably obesity – far more intensely than they do about celebrity gossip or even sports. Given the richness of the stories on these blogs, the Innovation Cell examines these stories on a regular basis to determine what people say they want out of their health care system. How, we wondered, do the obese and overweight say they *want* to be treated?

As we expected, the millions of personal weight loss stories described by individuals on the Web often tell highly specialized success tales that would not work for most people. These stories represent another rich source of weight-management information, different from that gathered by dieticians or doctors or research studies because they are self-reported and not told under the duress of sitting in the patient's chair. And in keeping with the message we have described in this book, the word 'fun' or 'enjoyable' pops up frequently in personalized accounts of successful weight loss and control.

The Innovation Cell's findings indicate that fun, 'low-tech' solutions to weight loss are the most frequently self-reported tools for success. This insight in no way disqualifies the value of medication or bariatric surgery for some, but it strengthens the policy argument in support of giving sufficient incentives for physicians and nurses to work with their patients to find out what sorts of things make for fun in their patients' lives, and prescribing an individual weight loss regimen that complements that activity. HLVs can then fund this 'trial of one.'

Unfortunately, the public health community does not value the 'trial of one.' It is often on the hunt for generic solutions that can be applied to all. And undoubtedly, some interventions – a pedometer, for example, since it is easy to meld into the everyday activities of busy people – suggest success at a population level. Consider a report published in November 2007 in the *Journal of the American Medical Association*: researchers at Stanford University analysed twenty-six studies involving 2,767 people and found that sedentary adults given a pedometer walked more than two thousand extra steps a day – roughly a mile – and lost weight.[170] However, these very same people who lost weight might each have a more individualized approach that could have worked better for them. As a matter of public policy, it is better not to bend to the bias of research that propels us toward cure-all policy solutions – for example, invest in free, fancy pedometers for all – versus policy solutions that allow providers to be better reimbursed for communicating candidly with their patients to design individual, sustained weight management solutions with HLVs.

Envoi

Shaming techniques, taxing the obese, and top-down messaging campaigns are ineffective, expensive, and reflexive ways to address the obesity epidemic. They do not work and they make many overweight people feel miserable. Yet policy people embrace them, and they remain popular with the public based on our global survey reported in this chapter.

We have seen how public health policy makers around the world increasingly believe that the power of shame can curb obesity. We have argued that such messages do not work. Worse, they are counterproductive: they introduce and reinforce dissatisfaction with body image, and they foster frustration and resignation.

The target of public health is the health of the community; the health of the individuals in that community is not the immediate concern. The distinction is important and potentially life saving. It matters for public health officials that the majority be healthy. Yet wrestling with one's weight always has been, and always will be, an intensely individual battle. The only meaningful public policy solution is to provide everyone, fat and thin, with direct financial incentives, and choices, to lead the healthier lives they want to lead. HLVs are one way forward.

Ecclesiastes 9:7. Go thy way, eat thy bread with joy, and drink thy wine with a merry heart.

Notes

1 SFGate, 'Could You Eat a Year's Worth of Grand Slams – If They Were Free?' http://www.sfgate.com/cgi-bin/blogs/dollarsandsense/detail?entry_id=59322.

2 C. Bacon et al., 'A Prospective Study of Risk Factors for Erectile Dysfunction,' *Journal of Urology* 176 (2006): 217–21.

3 A. Hammoud et al., 'Effect of Roux-en-Y Gastric Bypass Surgery on the Sex Steroids and Quality of Life in Obese Men,' *Journal of Clinical Endocrinology and Metabolism* 94, no. 4 (2008): 1329–32.

4 Columbia University Mailman School of Public Health, 'Obesity Now Poses as Great a Threat to Health as Smoking,' http://www.mailman.columbia.edu/research-service/obesity-now-poses-great-threat-health-smoking.

5 T. Pischon et al., 'General and Abdominal Adiposity and Risk of Death in Europe,' *New England Journal of Medicine* 359 (2008): 2105–20.

6 D. Campbell, 'Warning over Obesity in Pregnancy,' *The Observer*, http://www.guardian.co.uk/lifeandstyle/2010/jan/10/pregnancy-obesity-weight-mother-warning.

7 A.P. Polednak, 'Trends in Incidence Rates for Obesity-Associated Cancers in the US,' *International Journal of Cancer Epidemiology, Detection, and Prevention* 27, no. 6 (2003): 415–21. See also P.A. Van den Brandt et al., 'Pooled Analysis of Prospective Cohort Studies on Height, Weight, and Breast Cancer Risk,' *American Journal of Epidemiology* 152, no. 6 (2000): 514–27.

8 J.M. Petrelli et al., 'Body Mass Index, Height, and Postmenopausal Breast Cancer Mortality in a Prospective Cohort of U.S. Women,' *Cancer Causes and Control* 13, no. 4 (2002): 325–32.

9 A. Simpson, 'Cancers Caused by Obesity as Big a Threat as Climate Change,' *Telegraph*, http://www.telegraph.co.uk/health/health-

news/4781818/Cancers-caused-by-obesity-as-big-a-threat-as-climate-change.html.

10 M. Huckabee, *Quit Digging Your Grave with a Knife and Fork: A 12-Stop Program to End Bad Habits and Begin a Healthy Lifestyle* (New York: Center Street, 2005).

11 U. Keller, 'From Obesity to Diabetes,' *International Journal for Vitamin and Nutrition Research* 76, no. 4 (2006): 172–7.

12 F.M. Felicia et al. 'Ig2f Gene Variant and Risk of Hypertension in Obese Children and Adolescents,' *Paediatric Research* 67, no. 4 (2010): 340–4.

13 R. Poirier, 'Obesity and Cardiovascular Disease: Pathophysiology, Evaluation, and Effect of Weight Loss,' *Arteriosclerosis, Thrombosis, and Vascular Biology* 26 (2006): 968–76.

14 B. Liu et al., 'Relationship between Body Mass Index and Length of Hospital Stay for Gallbladder Disease,' *Journal of Public Health* 30, no. 2 (2008): 161–6.

15 F. Iannone and G. Lapadula, 'Obesity and Inflammation – Targets for OA Therapy,' *Current Drug Targets* 11, no. 5 (May 2010): 586–98.

16 Y. Chen et al., 'Increased Effect of Obesity on Asthma in Adults with Low Household Income,' *Journal of Asthma* 47, no. 3 (April 2010): 263–8.

17 S. Pandey and S. Bhattacharya, 'Impact of Obesity on Gynecology,' *Women's Health* 6, no. 1 (2010): 107–17.

18 A.M. Traish et al., 'Mechanisms of Obesity and Related Pathologies: Androgen Deficiency and Endothelial Dysfunction May Be the Link between Obesity and Erectile Dysfunction,' *Federation of Experimental Biological Societies Journal* 276, no. 20 (2009): 5755–67.

19 C.L. Fox and C.V. Farrow, 'Global and Physical Self-Esteem and Body Dissatisfaction as Mediators of the Relationship between Weight Status and Being a Victim of Bullying,' *Journal of Adolescence* 32, no. 5 (2009): 1287–301.

20 C.A. McCarty et al., 'Longitudinal Associations among Depression, Obesity, and Alcohol Use Disorders in Young Adulthood,' *General Hospital Psychiatry* 31, no. 5 (2009): 442–50.

21 L. Wang et al., 'Alcohol Consumption, Weight Gain, and Risk of Becoming Overweight in Middle-Aged and Older Women,' *Archives of Internal Medicine* 170, no. 5 (2010): 453–61.

22 T.M. Gadalla, 'Association of Obesity with Mood and Anxiety Disorders in the Adult General Population,' *Chronic Disease in Canada* 30, no. 1 (2009): 29–36.

23 G.E. Simon, 'Association between Obesity and Psychiatric Disorders in the U.S. Adult Population,' *Archives of General Psychiatry* 63, no. 7 (2006): 824–30.

24 S.L. McElroy et al., 'Are Mood Disorders and Obesity Related? A Review for the Mental Health Professional,' *Journal of Clinical Psychiatry* 65, no. 5 (2004): 634–51.

25 V. Marechal et al., 'Alexithymia in Severely Obese Patients Seeking Surgical Treatment,' *Psychological Reports* 105, no. 3 (2009): 935–44.

26 M. Kark, 'Obesity Status and Risk of Disability Pension Due to Psychiatric Disorders,' *International Journal of Obesity* 34, no. 4 (April 2010): 726–32.

27 K. Lazar, *Boston Globe*, 'Researchers Stress Fitness for Firefighters, EMTs,' http://www.boston.com/news/local/massachusetts/articles/2009/03/20/researchers_stress_fitness_for_firefighters_emts.

28 R.P. Wildman et al., 'The Obese without Cardiometabolic Risk Factor Clustering and the Normal Weight with Cardiometabolic Risk Factor Clustering,' *Archives of Internal Medicine* 168, no. 15 (2008): 1617–24.

29 Centers for Disease Control and Prevention, 'Overweight and Obesity,' http://www.cdc.gov/obesity/data/trends.html#State.

30 Centers for Disease Control and Prevention, 'Overweight and Obesity,' http://www.cdc.gov/obesity/stateprograms/fundedstates/new_jersey.html.

31 L. Trasande et al., 'Effects of Childhood Obesity on Hospital Care and Costs, 1999–2005,' *Health Affairs* 28, no. 4 (2009): 751–60.

32 Canadian Institute for Health Information, News Release: 'Health Care Spending to Reach $130 Billion This Year – Per Capita Spending to Hit $4000,' 8 December 2004.

33 A. Norton, 'All U.S. Adults Could Be Overweight in 40 Years,' *Reuters*, http://www.reuters.com/article/idUSCOL66909620080806.

34 M. Fox, 'Obese Americans Now Outweigh the Merely Overweight,' *Reuters*, http://www.reuters.com/article/idUSTRE50863H20090109.

35 '1.5 Million "Super Obese" in Canada, Mds Warn,' (2008). *Ottawa Citizen*, http://www.canada.com/ottawacitizen/news/story.html?id=98d1144a-7d8a-49fd-9b15-af31a4edcd18.

36 'A New Way to Combat Obesity,' *Manila Times*, http://article.wn.com/view/2006/12/15/A_new_way_to_combat_obesity, accessed 6 December 2010.

37 'Obesity Doubles in Sweden in 25 Years,' http://www.shortnews.com/start.cfm?id=60821, accessed 6 December 2010.

38 B. Butland et al. 'Tackling Obesities: Future Choices – Project Report,' *Foresight*, http://www.foresight.gov.uk/Obesity/17.pdf.

39 'African Obesity an Underestimated "Silent Killer,"' *Huffington Post*, http://www.huffingtonpost.com/2009/06/24/african-obesity-an-undere_n_220245.html.

40 'Does Size Matter in Africa?' *BBC News,* http://news.bbc.co.uk/2/hi/africa/4566870.stm, accessed 6 December 2010.

41 P. Zweck, 'I Wish Someone Would Do Something about How Fat I Am,' *The Onion,* http://www.theonion.com/articles/i-wish-someone-would-do-something-about-how-fat-i,11146.

42 'The World Health Organization Warns of the Rising Threat of Heart Disease and Stroke as Overweight and Obesity Rapidly Increase,' http://www.who.int/mediacentre/news/releases/2005/pr44/en/index.html.

43 S.J. Olshansky et al., 'A Potential Decline in Life Expectancy in the United States in the 21st Century,' *New England Journal of Medicine* 352, no. 11 (2005): 1138–45.

44 C. Burslem, 'Obesity in Developing Countries: People Are Overweight but Still Not Well Nourished,' http://www.worldhunger.org/articles/04/global/burslem.htm.

45 Oprah.com, 'When Oprah Met Bob,' http://www.oprah.com/health/When-Oprah-Met-Fitness-Expert-Bob-Greene/print/1.

46 N.A. Christakis and J.H. Fowler, 'The Spread of Obesity in a Large Social Network over 32 Years,' *New England Journal of Medicine* 357, no. 4 (2007): 370–9.

47 M.A. Pereira et al., 'Effects of a Low-Glycemic Load Diet on Resting Energy Expenditure and Heart Disease Risk Factors during Weight Loss,' *Journal of the American Medical Association* 292 (2004): 2482–90.

48 T. Philipson and R. Posner, 'The Long-Run Growth in Obesity as a Function of Technological Change,' *Perspectives in Biology and Medicine* 46, no. 3 (2003): s87–s107.

49 A. Ellin, 'What's Eating Our Kids? Fears about "Bad" Foods,' *New York Times,* http://www.nytimes.com/2009/02/26/health/nutrition/26food.html.

50 EurekAlert! 'Intellectual Work Induces Excessive Calorie Intake,' http://www.eurekalert.org/pub_releases/2008-09/ul-iwi090408.php.

51 M. Power and J. Schulkin, *The Evolution of Obesity* (Baltimore: Johns Hopkins University Press, 2009).

52 L. Cordain, *The Paleo Diet: Lose Weight and Get Healthy by Eating the Food You Were Designed to Eat* (New York: Wiley, 2002).

53 R. Audette, *NeanderThin: Eat Like a Caveman to Achieve a Lean, Strong, Healthy Body* (New York: St Martin's, 2000).

54 A. Stunkard, 'The Body-Mass Index of Twins Who Have Been Reared Apart,' *New England Journal of Medicine* 322, no. 21 (1990): 1483–7.

55 C. Bouchard et al., 'Overfeeding in Identical Twins: 5-Year Postoverfeeding Results,' *Metabolism* 45, no. 8 (1996): 1042–50.

56 N. Kurokawa et al., 'The ADRB3 Trp64Arg Variant and BMI: A Meta-Analysis of 44833 Individuals,' *International Journal of Obesity* 32, no. 8 (2008): 1240–9.

57 N. Ahituv et al., 'Medical Sequencing at the Extremes of Human Body Mass,' *American Journal of Human Genetics* 80, no. 4 (2007): 779–91.

58 H. Masuzaki et al., 'Augmented Expression of Obese (ob) Gene during the Process of Obesity in Genetically Obese-Hyperglycemic Wistar Fatty (falfa) Rats,' *FEBS Letters* 378, no. 3 (1996): 267–71.

59 R. Winslow, 'Genes Point to the Best Diets,' *Wall Street Journal*, http://online.wsj.com/article/SB10001424052748703862704575099742545274032.html.

60 Centers for Disease Control and Prevention, 'Obesity Still a Major Problem, New Data Show,' http://www.cdc.gov/nchs/pressroom/04facts/obesity.htm.

61 A. Mokdad et al., 'The Spread of the Obesity Epidemic in the United States, 1991–1998,' *Journal of American Medical Association* 282, no. 16 (1999): 1519–22.

62 D. Lakdawalla and T. Philipson, 'The Growth of Obesity and Technological Change,' *Economics and Human Biology* 7, no. 3 (2009): 283–93.

63 E. Finkelstein and L. Zuckerman, *The Fattening of America: How the Economy Makes Us Fat, If It Matters, and What to Do about It* (New Jersey: John Wiley and Sons, 2008).

64 S. Chou et al., 'An Economic Analysis of Adult Obesity: Results from the Behavioral Risk Factor Surveillance System,' *Journal of Health Economics* 23 (2004): 565–87.

65 P. Anderson et al., 'Maternal Employment and Overweight Children,' *Journal of Health Economics* 22 (2003): 477–504.

66 BBC, 'Obesity and Mental Health Linked,' *BBC News*. http://news.bbc.co.uk/2/hi/uk_news/scotland/8298080.stm.

67 L. De Witt et al., 'Depression and Body Mass Index, a U-Shaped Association,' *BMC Public Health* 9, no. 14 (2009).

68 C. Lliades, 'Foods That Fight Depression,' http://www.everydayhealth.com/depression/foods-that-fight-depression.aspx, accessed 6 December 2010.

69 S. Holt et al., 'A Satiety Index of Common Foods,' *European Journal of Clinical Nutrition* 49, no. 9 (1995): 675–90.

70 S. Luckhaupt et al., 'The Prevalence of Short Sleep Duration by Industry and Occupation in the National Health Interview Survey,' *Sleep* 33, no. 2 (2010): 149–59.

71 ScienceDaily, 'Reading Novel Can Help Obese Kids Lose Weight, Study

Shows,' http://www.sciencedaily.com/releases/2008/10/081004080918. htm. See also Beacon Street Girls, 'Meet Chelsea Briggs,' http://www. beaconstreetgirls.com/news-and-events/meet-chelsea-briggs.

72 M. Katz, 'I Put in 5 Miles at the Office,' *New York Times*, http://www. nytimes.com/2008/09/18/health/nutrition/18fitness.html.

73 InternetArchive.org, *Reefer Madness*, http://www.archive.org/details/ reefer_madness1938.

74 D. Kessler, *The End of Overeating: Taking Control of the Insatiable North American Appetite* (Toronto: McClelland and Stewart, 2009).

75 S. Vangala and A. Tonelli, 'Biomarkers, Metabonomics, and Drug Development: Can Inborn Errors of Metabolism Help in Understanding Drug Toxicity?' *American Association of Pharmaceutical Scientists Journal* 9, no. 3 (2007): E284–E297.

76 G. Wang et al., 'Evidence of Gender Differences in the Ability to Inhibit Brain Activation Elicited by Food Stimulation,' *Proceedings of the National Academy of Sciences*, http://www.pnas.org/content/106/4/1249.abstract.

77 Linda Brookes, 'Consciousness of Blood Pressure Is Rising: Cocoa-Rich Foods, but Not Tea, May Lower Blood Pressure,' 2007 Medscape Cardiology, http://cme.medscape.com/viewarticle/556658_5. Medscape login required.

78 L. Wang et al., 'Alcohol Consumption, Weight Gain, and Risk of Becoming Overweight in Middle-Aged and Older Women,' *Archives of Internal Medicine* 170, no. 5 (2010): 453–61.

79 T. Parker-Pope, 'Study Zeroes in on Calories, Not Diet, for Loss,' *New York Times*, http://www.nytimes.com/2009/02/26/health/nutrition/26diet. html?ref=us.

80 Christakis and Fowler, 'The Spread of Obesity in a Large Social Network over 32 Years.'

81 R. McKinnon et al., 'Considerations for an Obesity Policy Research Agenda,' *American Journal of Preventive Medicine* 36, no. 4 (2009): 351–7.

82 M. Schwartz and K. Brownell, 'Actions Necessary to Prevent Childhood Obesity: Creating the Climate for Change,' *Journal of Law, Medicine, and Ethics*, 35, no. 1 (2007): 78–89.

83 L. Baur, 'Tackling the Epidemic of Childhood Obesity,' *Canadian Medical Association Journal* 180, no. 7 (2009): 701–2.

84 H. Quartetti, 'Shedding Pounds for Life. Been There Done That. Successful Weight Losers Share Their Secrets for Keeping Weight Off for Good,' *Diabetes Forecast* 56, no. 4 (2003): 83–4.

85 Sheldon Margen Public Health Library, *What Is Public Health?* http://www. lib.berkeley.edu/PUBL/whatisph.html.

86 S. Satel, *PC, M.D.: How Political Correctness Is Corrupting Medicine* (New York: Basic Books, 2001).

87 R. McKinnon et al., 'Considerations for an Obesity Policy Research Agenda,' *American Journal of Preventive Medicine* 36, no. 4 (2009): 351–7.

88 M. Bittman, 'Soda: A Sin We Sip Instead of Smoke?' *New York Times*, http://www.nytimes.com/2010/02/14/weekinreview/14bittman.html.

89 FoodNavigator.com, 'Childhood Obesity on the Up in Sweden Especially in Girls,' http://www.foodnavigator.com/Science-Nutrition/Childhood-obesity-on-the-up-in-Sweden-especially-in-girls.

90 M. Fernandes, 'The Effect of Soft Drink Availability in Elementary Schools on Consumption,' *Journal of the American Dietetic Association* 108 (2008): 1445–52. See also E. Nagourney, 'Nutrition: Soda Ban in Schools Has Little Impact,' *New York Times*, http://www.nytimes.com/2008/09/23/health/nutrition/23nutr.html.

91 T. Parker-Pope, 'Hint of Hope as Child Obesity Rate Hits Plateau,' *New York Times*, http://www.nytimes.com/2008/05/28/health/research/28obesity.html?pagewanted=print.

92 J. Cawley, 'The Impact of State Physical Education Requirements on Youth Physical Activity and Overweight,' *Health Economics* 16, no. 12 (2007): 1287–301.

93 A. Krisberg, 'Institute of Medicine Plan Takes on Childhood Obesity: Major Recommendations Announced,' *Nation's Health*, http://www.medscape.com/viewarticle/492437. Medscape login required.

94 W. Saletan, 'Saturated Fat: The Genetic Limits of Obesity,' *Slate*, http://www.slate.com/id/2193026.

95 P. Anderson and K. Butcher, 'Childhood Obesity: Trends and Potential Causes,' *The Future of Children* 16, no. 1 (2006): 19–45.

96 C. Marcus et al., 'A 4-Year, Cluster-Randomized, Controlled Childhood Obesity Prevention Study: STOPP,' *International Journal of Obesity* 33, no. 4 (2009): 408–17.

97 J. Kropski et al., 'School-Based Obesity Prevention Programs: An Evidence-Based Review,' *Obesity* 16, no. 5 (2008): 1009–18.

98 QSRMagazine.com, 'The NPD Group Predicts a Change in Future Food Trends,' http://www.qsrmagazine.com/articles/news/story.phtml?id=8898.

99 T. Parker-Pope, 'Kid Goes into McDonald's and Orders ... Yogurt?' *New York Times*, http://www.nytimes.com/2009/06/16/health/16well.html.

100 MSNBC, 'As 23 States Get Even Fatter, Heavy Costs Loom,' http://www.msnbc.msn.com/id/31681795/ns/health-fitness/.

101 Mississippi Legislature, *House Bill 282*, http://billstatus.ls.state. ms.us/2008/pdf/history/HB/HB0282.xml.

102 S. White, 'Hotel Charges Fat Kids More for Their Lunch,' *Mirror News*, http://www.mirror.co.uk/news/top-stories/2008/08/23/hotel-charges-fat-kids-more-for-their-lunch-115875-20708260.

103 R. Kersh and J. Morone, 'The Politics of Obesity: Seven Steps to Government Action,' *Health Affairs* 21, no. 6 (2002): 142–53.

104 L. Gray, 'Fat People Causing Climate Change, Says Jonathan Porritt,' *The Telegraph*, http://www.telegraph.co.uk/earth/environment/climate-change/5436335/Fat-people-causing-climate-change-says-Sir-Jonathan-Porritt.html.

105 BBC News, 'Australia Airline "Fat Tax" Urged,' http://news.bbc.co.uk/2/hi/asia-pacific/7090529.stm.

106 J. Leeder, 'Fat-Guzzling Ads Not So Sweet,' *Globe and Mail*, http://www.theglobeandmail.com/life/health/fat-guzzling-ads-not-so-sweet/article1403444.

107 J. Scaperotti and C. De Leon, 'New Campaign Asks New Yorkers If They're Pouring on the Pounds,' NYC Health, http://www.nyc.gov/html/doh/html/pr2009/pr057-09.shtml.

108 N. Onishi, 'Japan, Seeking Trim Waists, Measures Millions,' *New York Times Asia Pacific,* http://www.nytimes.com/2008/06/13/world/asia/13fat.html.

109 M. Huizinga et al., 'Physician Respect for Patients with Obesity,' *Journal of General Internal Medicine* 24, no. 11 (2009): 1236–9.

110 D. Conley and R. Glauber, 'Gender, Body Mass, and Socioeconomic Status: New Evidence from the PSID,' *Advances in Health Economics and Health Services Research* 17 (2006): 255–80.

111 R. Puhl and C. Heuer, 'The Stigma of Obesity: A Review and Update,' *Obesity* 17, no. 5 (2009): 941–64.

112 H. Brown, 'For Obese People, Prejudice in Plain Sight,' *New York Times,* http://www.nytimes.com/2010/03/16/health/16essa.html.

113 K. Brownell and K. Puhl, 'Stigma and Discrimination in Weight Management and Obesity,' *Permanente Journal* 7, no. 3 (2003): 21–3.

114 Singapore-Window.org, 'Schools Making Fat Students Thin, But Emotional Burden Is Heavy,' http://www.singapore-window.org/sw05/050222a4.htm.

115 PRI's The World, 'Obesity Series Part III: Singapore,' http://www.pri.org/theworld/?q=node/14022.

116 R. Puhl and C. Heuer, 'Obesity Stigma: Important Considerations for Public Health,' *American Journal of Public Health* 100, no. 6 (June 2010): 1019–28.

117 S. Stewart et al., 'Forecasting the Effects of Obesity and Smoking on U.S. Life Expectancy,' *New England Journal of Medicine* 361, no. 23 (2009): 2252–60.

118 D. Albarracin et al., 'Immediate Increase in Food Intake Following Exercise Messages,' *Obesity* 17, no. 7 (2009): 1451–2.

119 G. Hirshey, 'Whole Grains, Fresh Corn: School Menu on a Mission,' *New York Times*, http://www.nytimes.com/2008/09/28/nyregion/connecticut/28colct.html.

120 ScienceDaily, 'Taxing Unhealthier Foods May Encourage Healthier Eating Habits,' http://www.sciencedaily.com/releases/2010/02/100224142046.htm.

121 P. Ubel, *Free Market Madness: Why Human Nature Is at Odds with Economics – and Why It Matters* (Cambridge, MA: Harvard Business School, 2009).

122 R. Rabin, 'Obesity May Have Offered Edge over TB,' *New York Times*, http://www.nytimes.com/2009/06/24/health/research/24fat.html.

123 A. Tucker et al., 'Prevalence of Cardiovascular Disease Risk Factors among National Football League Players,' *Journal of the American Medical Association* 301, no. 20 (2009): 2111–19.

124 Christakis and Fowler, 'The Spread of Obesity in a Large Social Network over 32 Years.'

125 'Comedian Ricky Gervais in Attack on the Overweight,' *The Telegraph*, http://www.telegraph.co.uk/news/newstopics/celebritynews/4076644/Comedian-Ricky-Gervais-in-attack-on-the-overweight.html.

126 BBC News, 'Obesity "Triggers" Disease Fears,' http://news.bbc.co.uk/2/hi/6921882.stm.

127 K. Harding and M. Kirby, *Lessons from the Fat-o-Sphere: Quit Dieting and Declare a Truce with Your Body* (New York: Perigee Books, 2009).

128 R. Puhl, T. Andreyeva, and K. Brownell, 'Perceptions of Weight Discrimination: Prevalence and Comparison to Race and Gender Discrimination in America,' *International Journal of Obesity* 32 (2008): 992–1000.

129 J. Latner et al., 'Assessment of Obesity Stigmatization in Children and Adolescents: Modernizing a Standard Measure,' *Obesity* 15, no. 12 (2007): 3078–85.

130 'New Survey Reveals Many Adults with High Cholesterol Fail to Take Necessary Steps to Improve Their Condition,' http://www.medicalnewstoday.com/articles/81501.php, accessed 6 December 2010.

131 M. Lindstrom, *Buyology: Truth and Lies about Why We Buy* (New York: Doubleday, 2008).

132 Ibid.

133 M. Flood, 'Some Experimental Games,' *Management Science* 5, no. 1 (1958): 5–26.

134 M. Jalonick, 'Michelle Obama Talks Anti-Obesity to Food Giants,' *MSN-BC*, http://www.msnbc.msn.com/id/35886607.

135 H. Wallop, 'Smaller Crisp Packets under Government Plans,' *The Telegraph*, http://www.telegraph.co.uk/health/healthnews/6702455/Smaller-crisp-packets-under-Government-plans.html.

136 A. Caban et al., 'Obesity in U.S. Workers: The National Health Interview Survey, 1986 to 2002,' *American Journal of Public Health* 95, no. 9 (2005): 1614–22.

137 S. Foerster, 'California's "5 a Day – for Better Health!" Campaign: An Innovative Population-Based Effort to Effect Large-Scale Dietary Change,' *American Journal of Preventive Medicine* 11, no. 2 (1995): 124–31.

138 F. Degnan, 'FDA's Recent Steps to Implement *Pearson v. Shalala*,' *Journal of American Nutraceutical Association* 3, no. 3 (2000): 3–5.

139 D. King et al., 'Adherence to Healthy Lifestyle Habits in U.S. Adults, 1988–2006,' *American Journal of Medicine* 122, no. 6 (2009): 528–34.

140 ConsumersUnion.org, 'New Report Shows Food Industry Advertising Overwhelms Government's "5 A Day" Campaign to Fight Obesity and Promote Healthy Eating,' http://www.consumersunion.org/pub/core_health_care/002657.html.

141 BBC News, 'Healthy Living Strategy Launched,' http://news.bbc.co.uk/2/hi/health/7204257.stm.

142 M. Dalton, 'Fighting Obesity May Take a Village,' *Wall Street Journal*, http://online.wsj.com/article/SB1000142405274870380890457452546271095 4426.html.

143 B. Montopoli, 'Senate Considers Federal Tax on Soda,' *CBS News*, http://www.cbsnews.com/8301-503544_162-5009316-503544.html.

144 S. Chan, 'NY Plan to Tax Soda a Bitter Pill for Some,' *New York Times*, http://articles.sfgate.com/2008-12-19/news/17133221_1_juice-drinks-obesity-american-beverage-association.

145 J. Pomeranz et al., 'Innovative Legal Approaches to Address Obesity,' *Milbank Quarterly* 87, no. 1 (2009): 185–213.

146 E. Gokcekus, J. Phillips, and E. Tower, 'Money, Race, and Congressional Voting on Vouchers,' *Public Choice* 119, nos. 1–2 (2004): 241–54.

147 N. Gillespie, 'The Father of Modern School Reform,' *Reason*, http://reason.com/archives/2005/12/01/the-father-of-modern-school-re.

148 C. Hepburn and A. Douris, 'Low Incomes, High Standards: Can Private Schools Make a Difference for Low Income Families?' *Fraser Institute*, http://www.fraserinstitute.org/search.aspx?searchtext=hepburn%20dour

is&folderid=145&searchfor=all&orderby=id&orderdirection=ascending&
LangType=1033, accessed 6 December 2010.

149 P. McEwan, 'The Potential Impact of Large-Scale Voucher Programs,'
     Review of Educational Research 70, no. 2 (2000): 103–49.

150 Dollarsfordieting.com, 'Dr Joseph Chemplavil – "dollar for pound" pro-
     gram news,' http://www.dollarsfordieting.com/in_the_news.htm.

151 Gillespie, 'The Father of Modern School Reform.'

152 Medical News Today, 'The U.K. Government's Obesity Initiative and
     Ill-Judged Partnerships with Companies That Fuel Obesity,' http://www.
     medicalnewstoday.com/articles/134924.php.

153 Docstoc.com, 'Where Science and Policy Meet,' *Conduit* 3, no. 3 (2009): 9.
     http://www.docstoc.com/docs/13618974/Conduit-Magazine-Fall-09.

154 CBC News, 'Survey Reveals Little Progress in Canadian Eating Habits,'
     http://www.cbc.ca/health/story/2009/10/19/consumer-nutrition-sur-
     vey.html.

155 R. Puhl, 'Obesity Stigma – Causes, Effects, and Some Practical Solutions,'
     Diabetes Voice 54, no. 1 (2009): 25–8. http://www.diabetesvoice.org/files/
     attachments/2009_1_Puhl.pdf.

156 D. Simmons, 'Citizen Journalism: School Vouchers at Risk,' *Washington
     Times*, http://www.washingtontimes.com/news/2009/nov/30/citizen-
     journalism-school-vouchers-at-risk.

157 L. Donnelly, 'Health "Voucher" for NHS Patients,' *The Telegraph*, http://
     www.telegraph.co.uk/news/uknews/1583294/Health-voucher-for-NHS-
     patients.html.

158 World Food Programme, 'WFP Launches First Food Voucher Operation in
     Africa,' http://www.wfp.org/news/news-release/wfp-launches-its-first-
     food-voucher-operation-response-high-food-prices-africa.

159 World Food Programme, 'WFP Launches Mobile Phone-Based Food
     Voucher Pilot for Iraqi Refugees in Syria,' http://www.wfp.org/news/
     news-release/wfp-launches-mobile-phone-based-food-voucher-pilot-
     iraqi-refugees-syria.

160 R. Smith, 'Obesity Crisis: Get Paid to Lose Weight,' *The Telegraph*, http://
     www.telegraph.co.uk/news/uknews/1576430/Obesity-crisis-get-paid-
     to-lose-weight.html.

161 h2cd.co.uk, 'Vouchers for Obese Who Lose Weight,' http://www.hc2d.
     co.uk/content.php?contentId=12030.

162 K. Junghyun and J. Herskovitz, 'South Korea Pays for Gyms for Obese
     Children,' *Reuters*, http://www.reuters.com/article/idUSSEO317338.

163 K. Volpp et al., 'Financial Incentive-Based Approaches for Weight Loss,'
     Journal of American Medical Association 300, no. 22 (2008): 2631–7.

164 R. Thaler and C. Sunstein, *Nudge: Improving Decisions about Health, Wealth, and Happiness* (New Haven: Yale University Press, 2008).

165 J. Bhattachrya and M. Bundorf, 'The Incidence of the Health Care Costs of Obesity,' *Journal of Health Economics* 28, no. 3 (2009): 649–58.

166 D. Saltonstall, (2009). 'President Obama Says "Sin Tax" on Sodas Is Food for Thought, Despite Gov. Paterson's Failed Proposal,' *New York Daily News,* http://www.nydailynews.com/news/politics/2009/09/08/2009-09-08_president_obama_says_sin_tax_on_sodas_is_food_for_thought.html.

167 A. Menendez, 'Voters versus Vouchers: An Analysis of Referendum Data,' *Phi Delta Kappan* 81, no. 1 (1999): 76–8.

168 C. Porter, 'Porter: How Sick Must You Be to Earn a Better Diet?' *Toronto Star,* http://www.thestar.com/news/gta/article/737921--porter-how-sick-must-you-be-to-earn-a-better-diet.

169 'New-Year Irresolution: How to Combat the Natural Tendency to Procrastinate,' *The Economist,* http://www.economist.com/business-finance/economics-focus/displaystory.cfm?story_id=15174430.

170 D. Bravata et al., 'Using Pedometers to Increase Physical Activity and Improve Health,' *Journal of the American Medical Association* 298, no. 19 (2007): 2296–304.

Index

The University of Toronto Centre for Public Management Monograph Series